Cases in
Long-Term Care Management
Building the Continuum

Cases in
Long-Term Care
Management
Building the Continuum

Edited by

Donna Lind Infeld, PhD
John R. Kress, MHA

Funded by a grant from
The Robert Wood Johnson Foundation

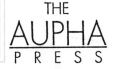

THE
AUPHA
PRESS

Published by
National Health Publishing
99 Painters Mill Road
Owings Mills, Maryland 21117
(301) 363-6400

A Division of Williams & Wilkins

The AUPHA Press is a joint venture between
the Association of University Programs in Health Administration
and National Health Publishing.

Printed in the United States of America
First Printing

Designer: Sandy Renovetz
Compositor: Absolutely Your Type
Printer: McNaughton & Gunn

Funded by a grant from The Robert Wood Johnson Foundation

ISBN: 0-910591-11-3
LC: 89-060-374

To my parents: Arthur, Arlene and Noah for
providing encouragement and long-term caring.
                                                    —DLI

To Anne: The girl I grew up with, the woman I'll
grow old with.
                                                    —JK

Contents

Part I. Introduction

Part II. Leadership and Management Decision Making

Part III. Operations

Part IV. Financial Planning

Part V. Strategic Planning and Community Relations

Foreword

Management is the foundation of every present or planned response to the challenge of providing appropriate long-term care. Appropriate care is not only humane for the individual and the community, but it is also cost-effective. As long as the long-term care sector remains dramatically undermanaged, many individuals and communities have little prospect of achieving appropriate care.

Undermanagement is the result of inadequate investment in managerial capacity, a shortage of professionally qualified health services administrators, and the managerial skill inadequacies of present administrators. There are many long-term care facilities and programs which are very well managed and stand out as such. They demonstrate the critical role of managerial competence in assuring the community appropriate long-term care.

Colleges and universities have an important role to play. This book is the product of faculty members from many schools working together to address the need for quality management training materials. The Association of University Programs in Health Administration, the consortium of academic centers for health management training, facilitated the book's development with support from The Robert Wood Johnson Foundation. This project demonstrates the potential of higher education in helping the community to achieve appropriate long-term care.

Gary L. Filerman, Ph.D.
President
Association of University Programs
in Health Administration

ix

Acknowledgements

Team work, group practice, collegiality, integrated efforts—these are common terms in education and the long-term care field. They are also particularly applicable to the process of developing a book. The editors are indebted to the sponsors, authors, advisors, writers, publishers, and production staff who collaborated to produce this casebook. We gratefully acknowledge:

- **The Robert Wood Johnson Foundation** whose generous support stimulated a wide range of programmatic efforts designed to expand interest and management competence in long-term care programs and facilities. This support included sponsorship of ten faculty fellows thereby broadening their exposure to long-term care settings. Special thanks to Jeffrey Merrill, Vice-President, who supported the publication of the case studies in book form.

- **Long-Term Care Faculty Fellows** who, chosen from among their peers at AUPHA member health administration programs, worked with executives in long-term care settings to gain an appreciation of current management concerns. They are the principal contributors to the casebook: William E. Aaronson, Heidi Boerstler, Diane Brannon, Richard L. Brown, Gary E. Crum, Seth B. Goldsmith, William E. Koprowski, Carlos A. Muñoz, Philip N. Reeves, and Henry W. Smorynski.

- **Long-Term Care Executives** who welcomed the faculty fellows, revealed their management problems, shared their administrative approaches, co-authored and reviewed drafts of several cases: Howard Braverman, Arturo Cadilla, Jr., Jared I. Falek, Elaine Frank, Jill Henson, Mary Hoffhaus, Eva M. Lauter, David Morely, Lin E. Noyes, Sylvia Schraff, David R. Seckman, Roy Smith, James F. Standish, Jr., Richard Wittenborn.

- **Task Force on Long-Term Care Administration Education** which guided the overall project and provided encouragement throughout this effort: Robert Burmeister, Joint Commission on Accreditation of Health Care Organizations; John Cornman, Gerontological Society of America; David Dunkleman, American

Association of Homes for the Aging; Elma Heidemann, Canadian Council on Health Facility Accreditation; Anne Katerhagen, National Association for Home Care; Paul Kerschner, American Medical Directors Association; David Kindig, University of Wisconsin; Philip Newberg, National Association of Boards of Examiners for Nursing Home Administrators; William Read, Hospital Research and Educational Trust; Richard Thorpe, American College of Health Care Administrators; Harvey Wertbleib, American Health Care Association.

Also contributing were staff representatives: Deborah Beitler, American Association of Homes for the Aging; Vera Reublinger, American Health Care Association; and Ann Tourigny, American College of Health Care Administrators.

- **Long-Term Care Administration Curriculum Committee** which established the criteria, selected the long-term care fellows, critiqued the book, and tested several cases in their classes: William Aaronson, Widener University; Bonnie Kantor, Ohio State University; Alma Koch, San Diego State University; Janet Reagan, California State University, Northridge; Raymond Rustige, St. Louis University; Cope Schwenger, University of Toronto; and David Smith, Temple University.

- **Barbara Buggele** who transformed endless drafts into text, charts, graphs, tables, and final copy, and never failed in enthusiasm and skill.

- **AUPHA Board and President, Gary Filerman**, for continuing to give priority to long-term care administration and establishing the Office of Long-Term Care and Aging as a vital unit within the Association of University Programs in Health Administration.

About the Editors

Donna Lind Infeld, Ph.D., is Associate Professor of Health Services Administration in the Department of Health Services Administration at the George Washington University in Washington, D.C. She has been educating long-term care administrators for over ten years. Her research has focused on quality of life in nursing homes, the impact of monitoring chronically ill patients on rehospitalization rates, and on utilization of hospice services. She is chairperson of the National Task Force and the Curriculum Committee of the Association of University Programs in Health Administration Long-Term Care Administration Education Project, funded by The Robert Wood Johnson Foundation to enhance curricula and provide support services to programs in expanding long-term care content and emphasis. Dr. Infeld has been a member of the Board of Examiners for Nursing Home Administrators for the District of Columbia, a fellow with the Accrediting Commission on Education for Health Services Administration, is an officer and fellow in the Gerontological Society of America and a member of the Research and Projects Committee of the Foundation of the American College of Health Care Administrators.

John R. Kress, M.H.A., is Director of the Office of Long-Term Care and Aging for the Association of University Programs in Health Adiministration in Arlington, VA. He is an experienced health administrator having worked as an executive of Family Health Care Inc., a leading consulting firm specializing in the development and management of primary care systems and programs both domestically and abroad, and HMO development. Other affiliations included a health planning agency, Regional Medical Program, cancer center development firm and a tour as a Commissioned Officer in the U.S. Public Health Service. More recently, he worked with Mountain States Health Corporation in Boise, Idaho on a Kellogg Foundation funded project to improve nursing home quality through the use of gerontological nurse practitioners in twelve western states. His current duties include the addition of long-term care related material in the curricula of health administration programs supported by a grant from The Robert Wood Johnson Foundation of which this volume is one product. Mr. Kress holds a Masters degree in Health Administration from Columbia University and a B.A. degree from the City College of New York.

Part I

Introduction

The Need for Leadership in Long-Term Care Administration

Donna Lind Infeld and John R. Kress

The aging population in the United States and Canada is a dynamic force altering the face of health and human services delivery systems (Infeld and Kress 1989). Stresses generated by the increasing number of elderly and other population groups needing long-term care services taxes these systems and stimulates new service structures, reimbursement mechanisms, and relationships among providers. Demand from the many organizations in the field for creative and effective executive leadership is great.

Long-term care embraces a broad array of services ranging from intensive and specialized geriatric screening programs to post-acute hospital care. It includes a host of institutionally-based medical and residential services, community-based services, and home care for those requiring medical care or assistance with activities of daily living. There are several definitions of long-term care:

> Long-term care consists of those services designed to provide diagnostic, preventive, therapeutic, rehabilitative, supportive and maintenance services in a variety of institutional and non-institutional settings, including the home, with the goal of promoting the optimum of physical, social and psychological functioning (Koff 1982, 3).

Koff (1988) recently suggested a more appropriate term would be *chronic care*, emphasizing the patient's needs, not the period of time involved. Evashwick (1987, 23) defines the continuum of care as:

> an integrated, client-oriented system of care composed of both services and integrating mechanisms that guide[s] and tracks clients over time through a comprehensive array of health, mental health, and social services spanning all levels of intensity of care.

While most cases in this book focus on one or two levels of care, they are generally concerned with issues of integration. According to Evashwick (1987, 3) there are four mechanisms by which services can be integrated: structure and organization, case management, information systems, and financing. These are recurring themes in the cases.

The growth in the number and complexity of long-term care service organizations has been dramatic, with projections for future expansion even greater. In spite of the resulting need for competent long-term care administrators, most health administration program graduates have been drawn to management practice in other settings. However, many factors previously perceived as deterrents to health care administrators entering the field of long-term care services are changing rapidly. First, the professional image of the long-term care administrator is improving. Salary incentives and benefit package levels have also become more attractive. Finally, as organizations increase in size and complexity, so do administrative opportunities. The demand for administrators with experience in long-term care services is also increasing in other health, housing, insurance, and related organizations as vertical integration and service diversification continue. The management challenges in care for the chronically ill require administrators to have firm grounding in management and strong executive leadership skills. Administrators must be effective managers to survive in this demanding arena.

Providing long-term care services offers qualified managers and administrators unique rewards, poses unique problems, and demands unique management skills. Administrators must appreciate, understand, and adapt to this uniqueness. The profession necessitates blending management and client interests. Meeting client needs and dealing with family and community scrutiny are considerably more demanding in long-term care than in other settings. The constantly changing, fragmented system of health, housing, and social services and the bewildering array of financing and reimbursement systems creates additional hurdles for administrators. Further, the intensity of services offered in nonacute settings is expanding rapidly. Nursing home and home health providers now deliver highly sophisticated medical care where once such services were found only in hospitals.

Long-term care administrators also face considerably different staffing patterns than do other health care administrators. Nursing home and home health agency directors must recruit, retain, motivate, and maintain quality personnel in the face of severe shortages of nurses and other professionals and high turnover in support staff often working in stressful environments. Long-term care directors generally work with fewer levels of management and professional staff than do their hospital counterparts. Nursing homes are heavily regulated now, and regulation may increase in other long-term care services as well, e.g., housing for the elderly, retirement communities, and home care.

General knowledge required to manage long-term care facilities and systems includes service coordination, clinical knowledge, social and community factors, law, ethics, management theory, supervision, system design, real estate, and others. More specific areas of knowledge include chronicity and its implications, geriatric assessment and care, characteristics of specific service settings, and family relations. Necessary administrative skills include management of finances, human resources, information systems, and complex systems arrangements. Thus, long-term care administration requires multiple levels of knowledge for effective management.

Providing long-term care is a management business but it is also a people business. Administrators are needed who can manage an array of services for the long-term care population. Executives should be disciplined and know how to manage, yet also be sensitive to the needs of the client, family and staff. They must be able to cross service lines and break traditional barriers in order to organize a continuum of care. The movement toward the development of a true continuum means that there are challenging opportunities for managers to shape the configuration of services and to influence the design of the service continuum of the future. A long-term care administrator is increasingly likely to work in an organizational structure that includes three or more service levels; e.g., elder housing, a skilled nursing facility, and home health and respite programs can be included on a single campus of care. Leading the development of a client-centered continuum is one of the most important challenges in health care today.

Use of Management Case Studies in the Continuum of Care

Donna Lind Infeld and John R. Kress

Fire!; financial shortfall!; to expand or not to expand?; How do we track our clients?—decision making is the major function of executives. Executives must lead, but how do administrators learn to make good decisions? One of the ways is to practice. The use of management case studies has proven to be an effective device to gaining decision making experience in an environment where errors are forgiven. In the real world, there is seldom a chance to experiment or to try again. The case method has been used for management education in university programs for many years (Andrews 1953). It has also been employed successfully by industry in corporate executive development and continuing education programs.

What is a Case?

The term "case" is used in many ways; e.g., patient case, law case. This book presents management cases—cases which describe a situation(s) or problem(s) faced by an administrator which requires analysis, planning a course of action, and decision making. The cases are designed to provide sufficient background information to understand the complex environment in which management problems occur; the student can then consider realistic options based on this information and the recommend a strategy to solve the problems.

Purposes of the Book

The goal of this book is to present a range of cases that assist the reader/student in developing or improving general knowledge of long-term care, management techniques, analytical skills, professional judgement, and personal values.

Knowledge. The cases present information about policies and procedures of various facilities, roles and responsibilities of staff, and characteristics of clients who use services. Cases are not designed to be the most efficient way to gain factual knowledge. Rather, they serve as vehicles to integrate knowledge gained through experience, previous reading and coursework. Situations and information presented in the cases should help students to synthesize experience, concepts, and theories. The process will also expand understanding of theoretical material.

Management Techniques. Cases provide the opportunity for students to apply techniques such as forecasting, budgeting, staffing, and strategic planning. Methods used by principals in the cases may be appropriate or inappropriate; the reader can evaluate the techniques which are used and apply others to the cases if they are more appropriate. In the case study method, deciding *when* to use a particular technique is generally as important as knowing *how* to use the technique.

Analytical Skills. Clear thinking, problem clarification, and sound decision making are extremely difficult skills to teach. A major benefit of the case study method is that it helps develop these particular skills. Cases simulate complex and ambiguous situations faced by administrators which often involve insufficient information, conflicting pressures, and often do not have a "right" solution. These situations require a decision, even if that decision is to take no action. After applying the appropriate analytical techniques to the situation, the reader must combine information, theoretical concepts, and common sense in a systematic process to reach a decision on how to proceed.

Professional Judgment. Optimal decisions require good judgment. It is essential to look at all sides of an issue, to minimize emotional reactions in the decision process, and to come to a decision that benefits clients and the organization. Professional administrators are distinguished by their ability to do this well.

Personal Values. Values are learned early in life and are difficult to change. Their influence and impact become apparent when examining decision-making processes involved in case situations. Organizational problem solving involves confronting the basis for and implications of decisions, and projecting expected consequences and weighing potential risks. In practice, the manager rarely faces a "win-win" decision. Through case study decision making, readers assess values and priorities that govern their decisions. The cases test the validity of personal values, and provide an opportunity to examine the consequences for their executive decisions.

Case studies are also excellent vehicles for building communication skills. Through both formal and informal presentations, participants gain experience in public speaking, quick thinking, and defending an analysis and resulting position. These are essential skills of the successful administrator. In formal educational programs, cases can be used to diagnose managerial weaknesses and develop new skills. In the corporate environment, cases can be used to sharpen skills, expand perspectives, and reinforce corporate culture.

How to Use the Cases

This case book is designed for use by two principal audiences. First, it can be used with upper level undergraduate or graduate students in health services administration, public health, gerontology, business, and nursing programs. Second, within the field of practice, it can be used by long-term care organizations and corporations in executive development and continuing education programs. The book can be used either in long-term care courses, in general health administration courses to provide long-term care material, or in "capstone" case studies courses. Cases can be used in lectures as reference points or examples. However, they are most often used with case method teaching where the responsibility of analyzing the case is left to students or participants.

There are two elements of the case method: Case discussion and case analysis. Case discussion changes participants from passive absorbers to active partners in dynamic learning. This process is not easy for participants or for instructors. It involves a new and democratic learning environment where participants must take responsibility for their own learning. For instructors, it involves controlling the temptation to give answers and direct the discussion in the typical patriarchical style (Andrews 1953, 7-8). Through case discussion, the group of participants develop, analyze, and debate various strategies for action. Participants take the perspective of the administrator or of a management consultant brought in to recommend optimal courses of action. Alternatively, participants can take perspectives representing the range of actors and interested audiences involved in the case. Whatever their perspective, they become decision makers in a real world situation.

Case discussions result in active learning. Participants must be prepared to get involved, feel what the administrator in the case is feeling, and examine how other participants might react. "We cannot effectively use the insight and knowledge of others; it must be our own knowledge and insight that we use" (Andrews 1985, 7).

Case analysis develops skills in written presentation and justifying a particular strategy. The process can take various forms. Basic steps in any analysis include:

1. *Analyze the case*: Prioritize relevant issues, players, and facts and identify missing information.

2. *Identify problems*: What are the fundamental problems or issues? Which are secondary? Are they controllable?

3. *Consider alternative courses of action*: Evaluate their strengths and weaknesses.

4. *Decide how to proceed*: Justify the decision and consider its implications.

There are no right or wrong answers. Some strategies are more promising than others. The important point is that a thorough analysis of the specific circumstances of the case is necessary in order to identify an optimum recommendation. All four stages of the analytical process are critical to the search for the best approach.

The Cases in This Book

These cases were written to present a range of long-term care settings and portray a variety of administrative problems and situations commonly encountered by their executives. They reflect many, but not all, levels in the long-term care continuum. The settings include skilled and intermediate care nursing care facilities, life care/continuing care retirement communities, hospitals, adult day care programs, home health care agencies, vertically integrated health care organizations, and community-based long-term care systems. The key decision maker is generally the administrator or chief executive officer. Other important managers include assistant administrators, directors of nursing, social workers, directors of dietary and housekeeping services, and long-term care consultants. Most of the cases were prepared by faculty members from the Association of University Programs in Health Administration member programs who worked with executives in the long-term care field to gain an appreciation of the management environment they face. Some cases use the real name of the facility and actual data in describing situations. In other cases, the organizational identity has been masked, yet the facts presented are based on true experiences and situations. A footnote to each case indicates their factual basis.

Some issues the cases address affect most long-term care settings. Examples include problems of staff turnover and recruitment, quality of care, reimbursement, and strategic planning. Other issues are more specific to individual setting types. For example, food service problems are specific to institutional settings. Each case reveals both general and specific issues. It is impossible to present all problems and situations confronting long-term care administrators. This collection presents a sampling of problems faced by practicing administrators and provides a sense of the variety of activities and problems which are part of the job.

The book of 14 cases is organized into five parts:

I.   Introduction

II.   Leadership and Management Decision Making

III. Operations

IV.   Financial Planning

V.   Strategic Planning and Community Relations

Cases are organized by the *primary* issue presented, however, most address multiple problems and issues. Some cases could have been placed in several sections of the book. Readers and instructors should consider all aspects of each case, not just the topic in which it has been categorized.

The cases can also be organized by service type and sponsorship. Since some of the organizations provide more than one service, cases fit into in multiple categories. Tables I and II can be used to help select cases according to sponsorship, service type, and residential setting. A separate volume, *Instructors Manual for Cases in Managing Long-Term Care Programs and Facilities*, is available to assist instructors using this book.

Conclusion

The variety of services and the issues faced by the administrators featured in these cases highlight important management challenges in long-term care administration. Strong and creative executive leadership for these diverse organizations is vital if new strategies

Table I-1 Cases by organizational sponsorship.

TITLE	Public	Non-Profit	Proprietary
		SPONSORSHIP	
ORGANIZATIONAL FAILURE	X		
FIRE!		X	
DIETARY DILEMMA		X	
TEAM BUILDING			X
RELOCATION		X	
DO NOT RESUSCITATE		X	
CLIENT DATA BASE		X	
CAPTURING LOST CHARGES			X
MARKETING & FINANCIAL		X	
COMMUNITY LONG-TERM CARE	X		
FINANCIAL CRISIS		X	
STRATEGIC PLANNING		X	
CONFLICTING STRATEGIES			X
CONTRACTUAL TIGHTROPE		X	

Table I-2 Cases by service location and level of care.

	LOCATION							
	IN-HOME SERVICES		COMMUNITY SERVICES		RESIDENTIAL SERVICES			
TITLE	Home Service	Home Nursing	Adult Day Care	Senior Center	Independent Living	Personal Care	Intermediate Care	Skilled Nursing
ORGANIZATIONAL FAILURE							X	X
FIRE!					X		X	X
DIETARY DILEMMA							X	X
TEAM BUILDING							X	X
RELOCATION							X	X
DO NOT RESUSCITATE							X	X
CLIENT DATA BASE			X	X			X	
CAPTURING LOST CHARGES							X	X
MARKET & FINANCIAL PLANNING		X						
COMMUNITY LONG-TERM CARE	X	X						
FINANCIAL CRISIS		X						
STRATEGIC PLANNING						X	X	X
CONFLICTING STRATEGIES		X				X	X	
CONTRACTUAL TIGHTROPE					X	X	X	X

are to both improve the quality of care for those in need and accommodate existing fiscal constraints.

References

Andrews, K.R., ed. 1953. *The case method of teaching human relations and administration.* Cambridge, MA: Harvard University Press.

Christensen, C.R. and A. Hansen. 1987. *Teaching and the case method.* Boston, MA: Harvard Business School.

Christensen, C.R., A. Hansen, and James F. Moore. 1987. *Instructors guide.* Boston, MA: Harvard Business School.

Evashwick, C.J., and L.J. Weiss. 1987. *Managing the continuum of care.* Rockville, MD: Aspen.

Infeld, D.L., and J. Kress. 1989 The Role of Health Administration in Services for the Aging: A exploratory look at supply and demand. *The Journal of Health Administration Education* 7(1):97-112.

Koff, T.H. 1982. *Long-term care: an approach to serving the frail elderly.* Boston, MA: Little Brown.

Koff, T.H. 1988. *New approaches to health care for an aging population.* San Francisco, CA: Jossey-Bass Inc.

McNair, M.P., ed. 1954. *The case method at the Harvard Business School.* McGraw-Hill.

Norville, Jerry L. A primer on case methodology and report writing. 1987. In *Instructors manual: Cases in health services management, second edition,* J.S. Rakich, B. Longest, and K. Darr, 149-150. Owings Mills, MD: AUPHA Press.

Penchansky, R., ed. 1968. *Health services administration: Policy cases and the methods.* Cambridge, MA: Harvard University Press.

Part II

Leadership and Management Decision Making

Introduction

Donna Lind Infeld

Several recurring themes emerge from the cases in this section. Administrators in every setting must make decisions about how to set goals, specify objectives, mobilize and motivate staff to achieve those objectives, evaluate results, and remain solvent or make a profit. There is a wide range of management styles that can be applied to these steps.

Factors important in making decisions appear throughout these cases. For example, long-term care administrators must take into consideration the extended relationship that their programs, and therefore staff, should have with clients. Continuity of care is particularly essential in nursing homes, adult day care centers, continuing care retirement communities, and to some extent, home health care agencies. Administrators must be aware of staffing patterns and characteristics which can interfere with this consistency and continuity of care. Therefore, hiring, firing, and motivating staff requires considerable administrative attention. On occasion, managers must hire people who lack optimal job qualifications. Nurses, of course, play critical roles in all long-term care settings and the director of nursing fulfills many important management functions as a key member of the management team. Several cases here and in other sections of the book address these human resources issues.

Managing relationships with a board of trustees or corporate directors demands considerable time and effort of most administrators. The goals of these governing bodies influence and/or determine the directions of the long-term care program or service. They serve a vital role in policy making which must be managed effectively to obtain optimal input from board members and prevent conflicts between the board and the department or program managers.

The first case, "Organizational Failure: Personal or Structural?" is set in a large county nursing home and as the case title implies, there are both structural and personal factors which result in violations of residents' rights and quality of care problems.

In "Fire!: Decision Making in a Crisis," most administrative decisions were made in the time frame of a few hours. However, the crisis experience suggests that plans were needed to address future emergency situations. The case setting is a continuing care retirement community.

"The Dietary Dilemma" focuses on decision making in the human resources area of a religiously affiliated nursing home. Hiring, firing, and contracting for services are decisions facing the administrator.

"Team Building at Carson Care," is set in a facility owned by a for-profit nursing home chain facing occupancy and financial problems. Several decision makers are involved in the case, but the administrator has the responsibility to take the initiative and get the organization to respond effectively to these problems.

In reviewing each of these cases, it is critical to keep in mind that the goal of the services being offered is to provide high quality care for elderly, chronically ill residents. Sometimes the details of operating an organization diverts attention away from this fundamental objective.

Case 1

Organizational Failure: Structural or Personal?*

William E. Aaronson

William E. Aaronson, Ph.D., is Assistant Professor, Department of Health and Medical Services Administration, Widener University.

John Willis strode over to the window of his office. The heat had become unusually oppressive for early June and John was already looking forward to some cooler weather. The heat that John was feeling was not just the warmth of a non-air conditioned office. His immediate superior, Robert Woods, had just left. John would be replaced as administrator of the Hidden Valley County Geriatric and Rehabilitation Center. An executive search would be initiated within the week. John would be staying on as the assistant administrator with responsibility for administrative support services, the position he had held until four years ago when he had become the acting administrator and, ultimately, the permanent administrator.

The History of the Hidden Valley Center

Hidden Valley Center is a 360-bed, long-term care facility that provides both skilled and intermediate care. Located in a suburban county of a major midwestern city, the center has a long, inglorious history. Founded as the Hidden Valley Almshouse in 1843 to serve the poor and destitute of the county, it was established as a working

---

* Fictitious names of both the organization and individuals are used to ensure anonymity.

poor farm for the unemployed in the local economy. In 1868, a large brick infirmary was built to handle the health care needs of the "inmates," many of whom were ill or disabled.

By the turn of the century, the center had become firmly established in the local community. The farm was self-sufficient and produced surplus crops that were used to feed the prisoners and orphans who were wards of the county. Over the ensuing decades, most of the residents of the home grew older and suffered from chronic illnesses and related disabilities. The center's role in the care of the frail elderly increased dramatically in the 1940s and 1950s as the impact of Social Security on the economic well-being of the elderly became more widespread.

By the 1960s most of the residents admitted to the center were old and infirm. The farm was worked by county employees rather than residents. County commissioners decided to sell some of the center's property and utilize the remaining grounds for county agency office space. Major building projects were initiated including construction of an office complex. The first modern nursing care building was erected in 1963. That building currently houses 120 beds.

The reputation of the center as a poor house is firmly established in the minds of the area residents, and the center continues to accept indigents only; even the road leading to the facility was named Poorhouse Road. With the advent of Medicaid in 1966, additional long-term care options became available to the poor and near poor. Private nursing care facilities opened as the Medicaid program rapidly became an important revenue source in the private nursing home industry. However, even with private options available through Medicaid, the need for the county nursing home continued to grow. The elderly population of the county was increasing rapidly, as it was elsewhere throughout the country. People seeking admission to Hidden Valley tended to be sicker and older, not poorer, than those entering private facilities, but only Medicaid-eligible applicants were permitted by county ordinance to enter the facility. This tended to perpetuate the poor house image of the nursing home since self-paying patients were not integrated with Medicaid patients as was customary in private nursing homes. The center grew, adding 120 beds in the 1970s and another 120 beds in the early 1980s. Occupancy rates consistently exceeded 98 percent. Six months ago, however, that growth changed.

Hidden Valley Center, like all county nursing facilities, is subject to political influence and control. However, the problems faced by

the center may have been much worse than in many other govern-
mental facilities because of political turmoil resulting from Valley
View County's strong two-party system. The center, as one of the
major human services budget items, had traditionally been a political
football. During the last election, the current county commissioners
had alleged that the previous board of commissioners failed to
exercise sufficient oversight of the center. They claimed that costs
had escalated too rapidly and that quality was declining. The
incumbent commissioners were defeated partly due to the elec-
torate's concern about the center.

Soon after the election, the administrator resigned. John Willis
was then appointed as the acting administrator while a nationwide
executive search was conducted. The hostile political climate in the
county and the low salary offered for the position impeded the
search. The county administrator, Robert Woods, concluded that
John was the best person for the job, and he was appointed as the
permanent administrator in 1984.

The Issue of Quality

Accreditation

Soon after becoming the administrator, John urged the county
administrator to free up additional resources that could be used by
the facility to seek accreditation from the Joint Commission on
Accreditation of Healthcare Organizations (JCAHO). Many staff
within the facility and at the county administrative level questioned
the value of accreditation for a county facility. The primary objection
raised was that there was no need to enhance market position since
they could not seek private paying clients. However, John felt
accreditation would enhance the image of the center and make it less
susceptible to political pressures at election time. The accreditation
process was long and arduous, but the objective of obtaining JCAHO
accreditation was achieved in late 1985.

The director of nursing (DON), Clara Higgins, expended
considerable time and energy on the accreditation process. She was
approaching retirement age and wanted to continue employment to
benefit from a generous retirement plan. However, she did not feel
she could continue to put forth the effort demanded of her position.
Even with JCAHO accreditation, pressure from the state department
of health was increasing. Quality of care in nursing homes had
become a major national issue following a report by the Institute of

Medicine, National Academy of Sciences, which found major flaws in the quality of the nation's nursing home system and made major recommendations for reform (Institute of Medicine 1986, 1-44). She knew that much more would be expected of the director of nursing in the next few years. She requested, and was granted, transfer to the position of Director of Education for the facility. A search was initiated for her replacement.

A New Director of Nursing with a New Priority

In the interim, a part-time evening nurse agreed to become the acting director of nursing. Joanne Simmons had recently returned to employment after raising her children. Although she lacked gerontological nursing experience prior to joining the center's nursing staff, she had been the administrator of a small intermediate-care facility for the mentally retarded and was a licensed nursing home administrator. The search for a DON was unproductive and Joanne was appointed as the permanent director.

Soon after her appointment, Joanne set as top priority greater recognition of residents' rights. No one contested the need to recognize the inherent dignity of each resident, but the floor nurses were still struggling to deliver an acceptable quality of care to their patients (Exhibit 1-1). They disagreed with the priority Joanne had assigned to residents' rights and felt that her idea of these rights was abstract and vague. The nurses were more concerned about difficulties in coordinating a care process that was hampered by absentee physicians and various center department staff whom the nurses felt were not cooperating fully with the nursing department personnel.

Nurse aides were also considered a problem by the floor nurses since aides received little or no direction and lacked initiative and enthusiasm in the care they provided. This lack of initiative was particularly troublesome for charge nurses on each floor since they lacked supervisory authority over nurse aides assigned to their floors. Each time a dispute arose between the charge nurse and a nurse aide, the shift supervisor had to intervene. Since shift supervisors had been assigned increased responsibility for clinical coordination and were required to ensure that physicians were providing adequate medical care, they had little time to provide direct supervision of the resident personal care performed by aides. Without supervisory authority, nurses felt powerless to correct poor technique or other case related activity.

<u>MEMORANDUM</u>

To: Clara Higgins, RN, Director of Education

From: Joanne Simmons, RN, Director of Nursing

Date: April 4, 198__

Subject: Item #21–Resident Privacy

The above deficiency cited by the state survey team indicates that nurse aides are not knowledgeable in the procedures of giving each resident a bath that allows for privacy and is done in an efficient manner. It is your responsibility as Director of Education to develop a reasonable policy in this area and provide inservice to the nurse aides on the proper procedure.

<u>MEMORANDUM</u>

To: Joanne Simmons, RN, Director of Nursing

From: Clara Higgins, RN, Director of Education

Date: April 5, 198__

Subject: Item #21–Resident Privacy

This deficiency is not the result of poor policy or lack of inservice. The nurse aides have received extensive training in this area. The problem is that they do as they please when the supervisor is not on the floor. The day that the survey team was there, the bathroom door was open and there was no visual privacy for the residents in the bathing room at the time. A directive from you and better supervision is all that is needed.

I will be glad to instruct your supervisors on management technique since this appears to be the source of many of the deficiencies.

Exhibit 1-1 Simmons/Higgins Memoranda.

The social services director, Scott McKenna, supported Joanne's stand on the issue of residents' rights. Together, they felt the image of Hidden Valley as a poor house had persisted too long and that the county commissioners had not done enough to change that image. They pressed their case with John. Essentially, they sought additional money from the county to improve environmental conditions and attain basic rights for the residents. For example, one recommendation was to install a telephone at each bedside so that residents would not have to rely on staff to assist with telephone calls. John agreed to assist with their efforts, but was reluctant to press the county for the funds to address all the deficiencies. The center's per diem costs were well above the state's Medicaid cost limits necessitating a county subsidy of between $1 and $2 million annually.

Joanne and Scott were not satisfied with John's response and promised further action if the issue of residents' rights could not be resolved to their satisfaction. Scott intimated that he was willing to take the issue to the press if he was not satisfied with the center's progress. He felt John was not sufficiently involved in the day-to-day operations of the facility and thought that he shared the same uncaring attitude about the center's residents as did the county Commissioners. Scott stated privately and publicly, on several occasions, that residents were considered second-class citizens and bore the historical stigma of poverty as residents of the "county poor house." He felt this image was unfairly and unnecessarily per-petuated and he was determined to change the image of the Center.

The Survey

The state survey agency recently adopted the new federal survey format for inspecting nursing homes. The Patient Care and Services (PaCS) survey was being implemented by the state to fulfill its commitment to ensure higher quality care in the state's nursing homes. In March, the state survey team visited Hidden Valley to conduct a totally unexpected survey initiated in response to a complaint lodged with the state survey agency. Hidden Valley experienced a PaCS survey for the first time. The surveyors began their visit on March 25.

The survey team did not find violations directly threatening the life or safety of residents. However, numerous deficiencies were found throughout the facility. Some deficiencies resulted from violations of residents' rights to privacy. They included bathing and dressing in view of other residents, staff, and visitors. Male residents were shaved in the hallway. Residents were bathed with a common bar of soap and many lacked personal toilet articles. Staff failed to receive adequate training regarding residents' rights and were not aware of the state's ombudsman program. Physicians failed to sign orders on several occasions. Maintenance work orders were not prioritized and work affecting resident safety or comfort were not given priority status. The center was cited for 28 deficiencies. The most serious, failure to manage, was levied because of the number rather than the gravity of any particular deficiency.

State surveyors also found Hidden Valley to be substantially out of compliance with standards and in violation of two federal Medicaid conditions of participation. The survey team leader expressed dismay over conditions at the center, since a full licensure survey completed just four months earlier at the center yielded only minor problems. The center was given 30 days to correct the deficiencies; fines were levied against it, and a process known as "fast-tracking," a compressed process for facility closure, was initiated.

The state survey team actions sent shock waves though the center and the county administration. Immediate action was required. With appropriate corrective action, the deficiencies could have been remedied easily. However, this was election year. Political ramifications made quick action even more imperative in an environment which would test the most seasoned administrator. Policy window

Management Response

The administrator held a meeting on April 1 with top management staff, including the director of nursing, the social services director, and 16 department heads, to discuss the center's strategy in responding to the survey results. The meeting was not productive. Most of the deficiencies cited crossed departmental lines. Each time an interdepartmental deficiency was discussed, department heads focused more on who was to blame rather than what should be done.

John Willis was most disturbed at the behavior of the director of nursing during the meeting. Joanne Simmons vociferously placed blame in three areas. First, she stated that the physicians were not sufficiently responsive to the medical needs of the residents. Joanne claimed to have interceded on several occasions to push attending physicians for appropriate diagnostic and treatment procedures when her floor nurses and supervisors had not been successful in convincing physicians of a resident's particular medical need. Second, she claimed that the maintenance department did not perform work in a timely manner. Further, she stated that the administrator had not supported her attempts to reform the nursing department. Finally, she explained that she would have been able to avoid the current difficulties if the administrator had recognized the critical importance of the nursing department and had granted her greater control over other departments, including clinical and nonclinical areas. John ended the meeting in frustration, but was determined to take the necessary corrective action.

Memo exchanges following the meeting failed to produce the spirit of cooperation required to resolve the inspection deficiencies and yield a full licensure status. Essentially, John requested that each department head develop remedial plans independently and report results to him. Memoranda between Joanne Simmons and Clara Higgins are indicative of the exchanges that took place following the April 1 meeting (Exhibit 1-1). John spent the next three weeks fighting fires resulting from the memo exchanges between department heads. On April 20, John sent a memorandum (Exhibit 1-2) to each department head. It resulted in a series of meetings between John and department heads, individually and jointly, which did not result in problem resolution.

The Surveyors Return

The state survey team returned on April 24 for a follow-up visit. Some deficiencies had been corrected, but the team found many new ones. The center appeared to be in a tail spin. John sought Robert Woods' assistance in analyzing and resolving the management problems that were resulting in the noted deficiencies. John and Robert met on April 28 to discuss the issues and to determine the next steps to be taken.

MEMORANDUM

To: Department Heads

From: John Willis, L.N.H.A., Administrator

Date: April 20, 198__

Subject: Responsibility for Plans of Correction

It has come to my attention that many disputes have arisen over responsibility for plans of correction. We have not corrected many of the deficiencies cited at the time of the last survey. I have attached a list of outstanding deficiencies which I had noted while making rounds. Each department head with some responsibility for the deficiency is to see me and explain the reasons for non-correction. I will then arrange for the department heads that continue to have disputes to meet with me together to resolve the dispute in my office.

Exhibit 1-2 Correction plans memorandum.

The County Administrator

Woods was determined to get to the bottom of this problem. He was responsible for the supervision of all county functions, excluding the court system. There were many issues in other county departments which had kept him from spending as much time at the center as he would have liked. Robert enjoyed visiting with the staff and residents of the facility. It was a pleasant change from his other responsibilities. The prison had undergone considerable turmoil resulting in the resignation of the warden. The county highway system had not kept up with the rapid growth and transition from a rural to suburban county. In general, Robert experienced increased difficulty maintaining the quality of county services in an environment of shrinking federal assistance and county taxpayers unwilling to bear an increasing share of the financial burden for programs. Consequently, Woods had not given the center much attention. After JCAHO accreditation was received, he reasoned that close scrutiny of facility operations was no longer necessary. Cost overruns were common at the center, but costs in general had not increased as rapidly as those of other county services.

To Robert, John appeared to be doing a credible job. County commissioners received relatively few complaints about conditions at the center; newspapers had not run a front page story on the center for two years; and the state nursing home ombudsman had not received any substantive complaints from residents or families. Finally, union activities were noncombative compared with other county departments. Robert would have gladly presented the same type of report that he had about the Hidden Valley Center to the county commissioners for each of his departments. Consequently, the state survey results were particularly troublesome to Robert. He decided that his direct intervention into the center's operations was unavoidable.

Robert identified three areas that would require investigation. First, he reviewed the organizational structure. Second, he reviewed existing policies and procedures, and finally, he initiated interim performance ratings for all managers. The first and third tasks caused Robert the most concern.

The administrative organization of both the center as a whole and the department of nursing were carefully scrutinized (Exhibits 1-3 and 1-4, respectively). In reviewing the organization of the center, Robert noted that 21 department heads and four staff level positions reported directly to the administrator. Robert reflected on his

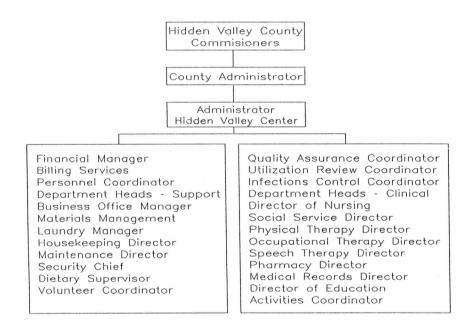

Exhibit 1-3 Hidden Valley Center Organization Chart.

decision not to retain John as Assistant Administrator for Support Services. When John was finally promoted to permanent administrator, the move saved money for the county, and John seemed able to handle operations without an assistant; this, Robert thought, avoided the need for position approval within the county which was extraordinarily cumbersome.

Prior to 1984, the administrator was a registered nurse. She had responsibility for all clinical services and delegated responsibility for all support services to John, her assistant. When the former administrator resigned, Clara Higgins, as director of nursing, had assumed responsibility for most of the clinical services since John lacked experience supervising health related professionals. John's undergraduate degree was in business administration. Clara held a master of science degree in nursing with a clinical specialty in gerontological nursing. When Clara received her requested demotion, Robert trusted John's judgement and had not questioned the issue of Joanne's appointment. Since Joanne's experience in gerontological nursing was limited, she was not given the added responsibility of supervising non-nursing clinical departments.

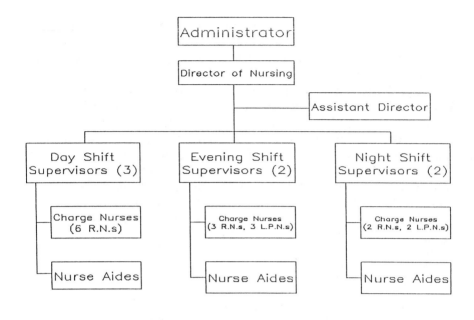

Exhibit 1-4 The Department of Nursing Organization Chart.

After intense review of the center's organization and its precarious situation, Robert decided that John needed immediate assistance to avoid the danger of closure. Robert assumed all routine operational responsibilities so John could concentrate on eliminating the deficiencies cited. In an attempt to resolve the center's administrative problems and to convince the state survey agency that the county was committed to full compliance with federal and state regulations for nursing homes, Robert initiated a study to determine the appropriate organizational structure for the facility. He also initiated performance evaluations of the administrator and director of nursing. — systems not Personnel

The evaluations were the more important tasks for two reasons. First, Robert could assist John and Joanne identify personal performance problems, and second, he could use the performance evaluations as a basis for improvements. If necessary, Robert would also have sufficient documentation to discharge them; he considered doing that as an immediate response to the crisis. However, documentation of previous performance problems was completely lacking. John had not been evaluated since he assumed his current position and he had just initiated an interim evaluation of Joanne due to the poor performance of the nursing department during the recent surveys. Joanne's previous evaluation, completed in September, 1986, indicated that she was doing an acceptable job as the director of nursing.

The complexity of administrative due process as defined in the state's civil service act inhibited personnel actions against Joanne. A civil service employee could be summarily dismissed for gross insubordination or seriously jeopardizing the health and safety of fellow employees or clients. Termination for poor performance required extensive documentation. In February, John requested assistance from Robert in firing Joanne and replacing her on an interim basis with Clara Higgins. Clara would have accepted the position earlier but was unwilling to accept the position under the present circumstances.

The Memo

Robert was also concerned about employee loyalty. The conflict between John and Joanne over residents' rights could have become an even greater problem if the press had reported the issue. The minority political party might also have used it for political gain. Robert's greatest fears were affirmed when a memo from Scott McKenna appeared on every bulletin board of the facility and on the editorial page of the county's largest newspaper (Exhibit 1-5).

Robert's immediate response was to fire Scott for gross insubordination and incitement of fellow employees. He felt this action was justified given Scott's blatant disregard for normal reporting channels. The action was supported by each of the county commissioners, including the minority members. This incident increased Robert's resolve to take quick action to curtail further deterioration of the present situation. The week following the firing was filled with meetings between Robert and several of the key management staff members. By the end of the week, Joanne had tendered her resignation. Robert appointed Ann Smith, Assistant Director, as the acting director of nursing.

Robert was still reluctant to take any action against John since it now appeared that conflict would be reduced in the absence of Joanne Simmons and Scott McKenna. Ann Smith had considerable experience in gerontological nursing in both nursing home and hospital settings. Robert had confidence that most problems would be resolved before the next survey team visit.

MEMORANDUM

To: County Commissioners

From: Scott McKenna, Director of Social Services

Date: May 6, 198__

Subject: Violations of Residents' Rights

As you are aware, Hidden Valley Center has been found to be in violation of State and Federal Statutes regulating nursing homes. The State Survey Team has found the Home to be deficient in several areas directly affecting patient care. I have made a good faith effort to work with the Administrator over the past six months to alleviate the conditions which resulted in the cited deficiencies. However, the Administrator has been either reluctant or incapable of addressing the very basic issue at stake here. That issue is one of residents' rights. Following the recent surveys, the Administrator has demonstrated that he is insensitive to both residents and employees. The time has come for John Willis to step down from the position of Administrator. Failure to take the appropriate action will only serve to perpetuate the problem since the State Survey team will not tolerate the continued violation of Residents' Rights and the County should not either.

Exhibit 1-5 Patient's rights memorandum.

The Next Survey Team Visit

On May 28, the survey team appeared in John's office at 8:00 A.M. Much to John's pleasure, many of the deficiencies had been resolved, a few still required action, but no new deficiencies were cited. Those remaining did not jeopardize resident health or safety and, with the progress made, the survey team announced that the center would receive a six-month provisional license. Management would have to send bimonthly progress reports to the survey team supervisor and an interim inspection would be required to oversee the progress made in correcting outstanding deficiencies.

During the visit, the survey team met privately with Robert to discuss the progress the center had made and to secure the county's commitment to full compliance with regulations. During the discussion, the survey team leader expressed concern over John's leadership ability. She focused on his unfamiliarity with clinical areas and stated that, although it is not necessary for the administrator to be a clinician, it was important for the administrator to be knowledgeable about patient care.

The Decision

Following the survey team visit, Robert realized what the problem had been all along. He decided to meet with John early the following week. It was difficult for Robert to accept that John would not succeed as the administrator unless he expanded his awareness of patient care. Robert could not risk John's continued failure to grow in this area, but he viewed John as a valuable employee and did not want to fire him. John could fill the management void by assuming his former position as Assistant Administrator for Support Services. The search for a new administrator would begin immediately.

Reference

Institute of Medicine. 1986. *Improving the quality of care in nursing homes.* Washington, DC: National Academy Press.

Case 2

Fire!: Decision Making in a Crisis*

Donna Lind Infeld and Eva M. Lauter

Donna Lind Infeld, Ph.D., is Associate Professor, Department of Health
Services Administration, School of Government and Business Administration,
The George Washington University, Washington, D.C.

Eva M. Lauter, M.S.N., NHA, is the Administrator of a life care facility in
Washington, D.C.

The Christian Home of Williamstown was organized in early
1890 by the Christian Churches of New Columbia. The purpose of
the home is to provide a comfortable residence with medical and
other necessary support for the aged members of the Christian
Church.

The home offers life care services with intermediate and skilled
nursing units. Affirmation, understanding, and the care of persons
over 65 in a Christian spirit is the philosophy of the home's program.

The home is overseen by a board of trustees composed of five
prominent businessmen with hospital management experience. In
addition, a board of managers made up of 85 volunteer members is
charged with general management. A nine member executive
committee of this board is actively involved in the operations of the
facility. The administrator, Mrs. Evans, licensed by the state, is in
charge of the day-to-day activities. Exhibit 2-1 illustrates the
organizational structure of the home.

---

* Parts of this case were first reported in *Housing the Elderly Report*, Silver Spring, M.D.,
September 1987. The names and places in this case are fictional.

Services Offered

The home has 51 independent living units and a nursing center with 26 licensed beds. Each independent living unit consists of a one-room apartment with a private bath. Residents in the independent living units can decorate their apartments with their own furniture. In fact, many of the residents have rooms filled with valuable antiques. All meals are communal for residents of the independent living units. The nursing center includes two skilled care beds and 24 intermediate care beds. It is important to note that the nursing center and independent living units of the home operate under different sets of rules and legal requirements. For example, the rules for marking fire extinguishers and exits are more extensive, and the requirements for staff training about emergency procedures are more detailed for the nursing care unit than for the independent living units.

Applicants for admission to the home must be at least 65 years of age, of good health and character, and a member in good standing of a Christian Church in New Columbia for at least two consecutive years immediately before application and be recommended by the pastor and officers of the advisory board. Residents range in age from their 80s to over 100 with a mean age of 87. There are 72 women and five men.

The home is concerned with both the physical and emotional well-being of residents, and recognizes that the elderly, as all other age groups, have a variety of needs to be met. Thus, the home is concerned with the whole person, and so provides basic services for housing, food, security, temporary and long-term intermediate and skilled nursing care, companionship, the promotion of self-esteem, and opportunities for personal and spiritual growth.

Staffing

The philosophy of the home includes the expectation that staff will care for and support residents with the highest degree of dedication, and treat them with respect and dignity in the same way in which they would expect to be treated by all of the others in the home.

Several key staff members fill important roles in the safe operation of the home: the administrator, the director of nurses, the food service manager, and the engineer.

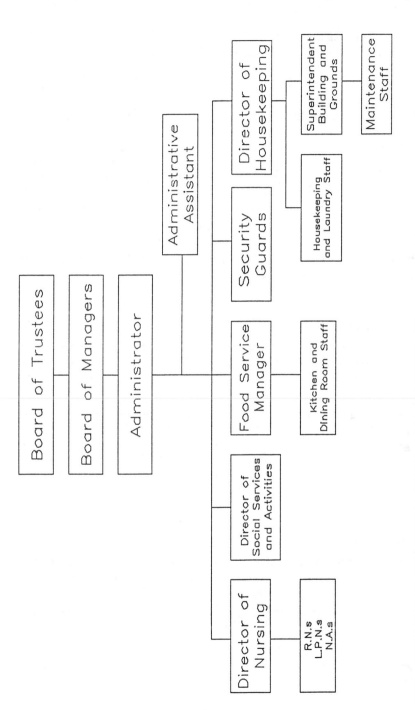

Exhibit 2-1 The Chrisitian Home of New Columbia Organization Chart.

The administrator, Mrs. Evans, came to the home four months ago. After eight years of experience in hospital and public health nursing, she completed post-graduate work in long-term care administration at the New Columbia State University. The home required that, as administrator, she maintain a room in the independent living section of the building and stay there at least five nights a week.

The director of nurses (DON) had only been at the home for six months. All of her previous experience had been in hospital settings. Whereas she had good working relations with the nursing staff, Mrs. Evans felt that the DON was not good at delegating responsibility.

The food service manager had been with the facility for two years, but had 20 years of experience in long term-care facilities. The engineer had 40 years of experience, including six years at the Christian Home. Typical staffing for the home for all three shifts (day, evening, night) is shown in Table 2-1.

Physical Structure of the Home

The two-story building was erected and dedicated in November 1924. In 1963 a new wing was built to house more residents. The building has the feeling of a grand mansion, with its stained wood trim and furnishings of period antiques.

Exhibits 2-2, 2-3, and 2-4 show the layout of the first floor, second floor, and basement of the building respectively. There is also a large attic. The administrator's office, library, dining room, and lounge are all on the first floor. Independent living rooms are on both floors and the entire nursing center is located on the second floor toward the rear of the building.

The Fire Safety Plan

The procedures for fire and disasters are described in the employee handbook of the home. Each employee is to receive, read, and understand a copy of the fire evacuation plan at the time of employment. The plan, also posted in the halls of the home, was approved in 1961, 1971, and 1982 by the Williamstown Fire Department.

Table 2-1 Staffing for the Christian Home of Williamstown

Shift/Dept.	Staff	Total Staff
Day shift (7:00 A.M. to 3:00 P.M.)		
Administration	Administrator, administrative assistant, part-time secretary	3
Food service	Food manager, 2 cooks, 5 waitresses, utility man	9
Nursing service	Director of nurses, day charge nurse, L.P.N., 5 nursing assistants	8
Housekeeping	Supervisor, 7 housekeepers, houseman, engineer, assistant engineer	11
	Total	31
Evening shift (3:00 P.M. to 11:00 P.M.)		
Administration	Administrative assistant (until 6:00 P.M.)	1
Food service	Cook, utility man, 4 waitresses	6
Nursing service	R.N., 2 nursing assistants	3
Security	Guard	1
	Total	11
Night shift (11:00 P.M. to 7:00 A.M.)		
Nursing service	R.N., 2 nursing assistants	3
Security	Guard	1
	Total	4
	Total staff	46

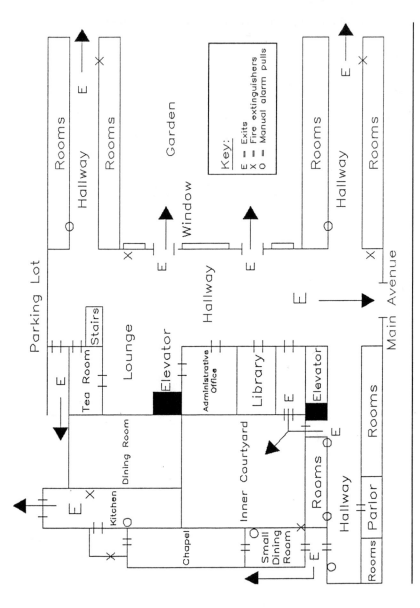

Exhibit 2-2 First floor fire emergency layout.

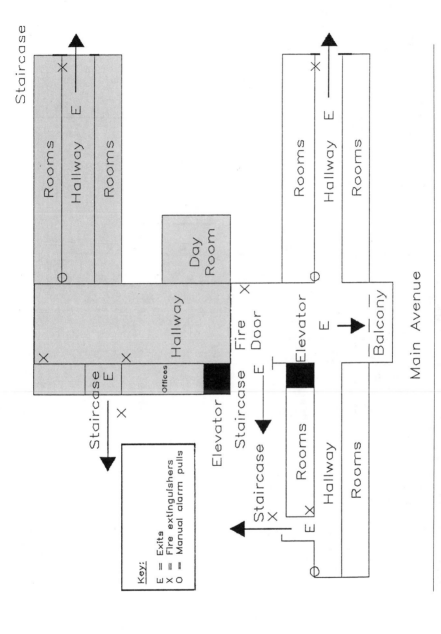

Exhibit 2-3   Second floor fire emergency layout. The Healthcare center is represented by the screened area.

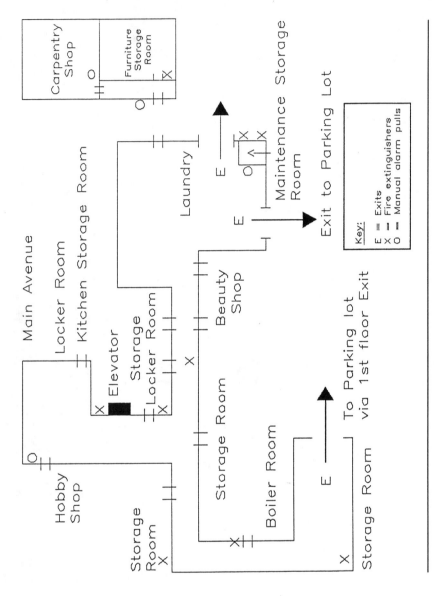

Exhibit 2-4 Basement fire emergency layout.

Employees are given the following instructions:

If you notice a fire or any other impending disaster, immediately:

1. Rescue residents from imminent danger. Leave them in their rooms to await instructions.

2. If it is a fire, confine it by closing the door of the room where you detect the smoke or flames.

3. Sound the alarm at the nearest alarm station.

4. Secure the area. Close doors, windows, and shut off electrical, gas, and oxygen equipment in the vicinity of the fire unless you and others are endangered.

5. If the fire is small, use the nearest fire extinguisher. Again, do not endanger yourself or others.

6. Contact the administrative office or the charge nurse on duty in the health center for further instruction.

The home tests the evacuation plan at unscheduled intervals. As required by the Medicare Conditions of Participation, a surprise drill is held for each shift at least quarterly. During the drill, staff members close all fire doors, move residents to safe areas, and await further instruction. Full evacuation is not required. During annual inspections, the fire chief noted only one deficiency: the time limit for inspection of some of the fire extinguishers had expired.

The Fire

On August 15, painters were working on restoring the wood entrance of the Christian Home. A blowtorch was being used to remove some of the old paint. The torch had set off the fire alarm connected to the fire station twice that morning, therefore, the alarm system was temporarily inactivated. When the painters stopped work for lunch, a breeze fanned the hot wood into a blaze. At 1:10 P.M., a passenger on a city bus saw fire and smoke coming out of the front of the home. She got off the bus, ran into the building, and warned a staff member who was on duty in the lobby. Since the flames were coming out of the outer portico on the second floor of the building, no one inside was aware of it. The staff member called the fire department and informed the administrator.

When the fire broke out, Mrs. Evans was eating in the downstairs dining room with the independent residents. She rushed outside, saw the extent of the blaze, returned, and ordered an immediate evacuation of the dining room through the nearest exit into the garden. Staff took control and residents were not permitted to go to their units for bank books, valuables, or any other reason.

Mrs. Evans then rushed upstairs and found smoke in the upstairs hall in the front of the building. The building did not have a sprinkler system (it was approved for occupancy based on a grandfathering provision for existing facilities), so the fire was spreading fast. Meanwhile, the most disabled skilled nursing residents, eating in the day room behind tight-fitting metal fire doors, were unaware of the fire. The director of nurses was there, along with two R.N.s, one L.P.N., and five aides.

Three residents were being fed in their rooms, and Mrs. Evans ordered them brought to the day room. Most were already in wheelchairs, but the rest were put in chairs from the adjoining storeroom. Since elevators are not used during a fire, Mrs. Evans told the group to wait in the day room, pending further instructions.

The home's emergency plan calls for residents to be put in their rooms in a fire situation, to await evacuation. However, with everyone already gathered in two places, Mrs. Evans decided to override the plan to keep better control and speed the removal of the patients to safety.

With a fire station across the street, firemen were on the scene in about five minutes. Because a "Code 4" alarm designates the location as a nursing home, over 30 fire trucks responded to the fire. The fire chief ordered those nursing center residents gathered in the day room moved to the end of the hall away from the fire and covered with sheets and blankets. Aides and nurses wheeled them there, explaining only, "We have to go down the hall now," without saying anything about the fire. Many of the nursing center residents are normally quite confused, but there was no panic. One aide reassured a patient, saying it was "only a drill."

Staff members began to transfer the residents to sheets and to slide them down a narrow back stair. There was some concern about injury, because of their frailness. After nursing personnel had moved three residents down the stairs, firemen came and carried the rest down in their arms. Health center residents were laid on sheets and pillows on the ground just beyond the stairwell exit. The ground was hard; without much padding on their bodies, the residents groaned from discomfort. Aides used wet cloths to cool the residents' faces and necks. Mrs. Evans checked their condition and had a small oxygen tank brought out as a precaution.

Meanwhile, in the garden, the independent residents from the dining room were put in chairs under the trees, and kept together as a group. At this point, Mrs. Evans rushed to her office to get the resident roster so she could make sure that everyone was out of the building.

The worst part was the weather. It was 95 degrees and very humid, as Williamstown often is in August. The fire department brought a service vehicle which supplied cool drinks, and the ambulance crews were there if needed.

The fire crews took hoses down the length of the first floor hall and up the stairwell in the back of the building. This was necessary because the wind was coming from the direction of Main Avenue, and it was necessary to spray water toward the wind. Details of the location of the fire are shown in Exhibits 2-5 and 2-6. The fire chief set up his command post, with walkie-talkies, outside the front door. When the fire chief needed to know the location of the electrical control panel for the building, the engineer was nowhere to be found.

In addition to firemen, ambulance crews, and police, the press arrived during the crisis. Two television stations sent mobile cameras, and the reporters, who seemed to be everywhere, were constantly putting the microphone in front of Mrs. Evans and requesting comments at very inopportune times. In a state of frustration, Mrs. Evans finally asked the fire chief to get the press to leave. It was hard to answer their questions in the midst of a crisis. Adding to the confusion were neighbors from nearby apartment buildings who rushed to the scene to help out.

A head count on the lawn confirmed that everyone was accounted for, but the fire chief insisted on checking the building to make sure. The only creature they discovered still inside was Mrs. Evans' dog, in her room.

Meanwhile, outside on the lawn, there was still uncertainty. Firemen with hoses were still fighting the fire. Mrs. Evans had established a control center in her office from which she had a clear view of the residents outside in the garden yet her office was well away from the fire area. The director of food service was at the control center to help out. Mrs. Evans called a nearby nursing home with whom she had emergency back-up arrangements and asked its

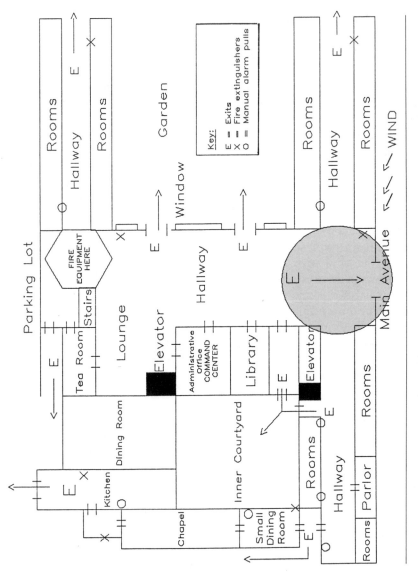

Exhibit 2-5 First floor fire emergency layout. The damaged location is represented by the screened area.

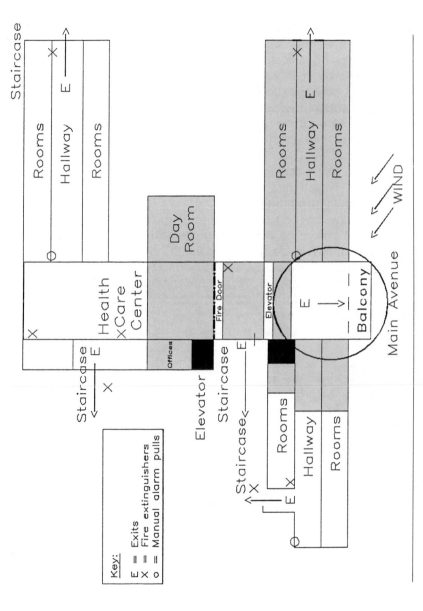

Exhibit 2-6 Second floor fire emergency layout. The damaged location in represented by the screened area. The fire is in the circled area.

administrator if 15 beds could be set aside for possible use that night. He agreed and in addition to preparing cots in hallways and extra food for the special diet needs of the residents, he asked his staff to work overtime, and dispatched a station wagon, nurses, and aides to help care for the Christian Home residents.

The fire was out by about 3:30 P.M. However, the building was not declared safe for occupancy by the fire chief until all smoke had cleared, more than an hour later. The standby beds at the other home were not needed. The kitchen was intact, so meals could be served. Since lunch was interrupted, the residents were hungry and were given refreshments and juice in the dining room as soon as they could enter the building.

The damage to the residents' rooms included six doors knocked down by firemen during the search for additional residents when the master key didn't work quickly enough. Nine independent living rooms and four health center rooms were damaged by water. While there was some damage to residents' personal belongings, it was generally covered by individual insurance policies. The home was not responsible for personal property.

In addition, the offices and the day room in the health center were damaged. There was substantial damage to walls, ceilings, furniture, rugs, and electrical fixtures due to the enormous amount of water sprayed into the attic; the fire damaged the porch, roof, and attic. Exhibits 2-5 and 2-6 show the damaged areas of the building.

At 6:30 P.M. the local nursing home inspector called to find out the extent of the damage. He had heard about the fire on the news and wanted to know how many units were affected and what was being done to take care of the residents. About an hour later the inspector arrived to check on the situation and to offer assistance.

Residents whose rooms were not damaged moved back in to sleep in their own rooms that night. Fortunately, there was room for residents of damaged rooms to stay in the facility too. In the nursing care center four beds were available. In the main part of the home there are three rooms normally available for guests. Several residents moved into these rooms and two others voluntarily chose to stay with friends or family members. These temporary arrangements were necessary for the following two weeks.

After the fire crews left, there were still problems to resolve. Parts of the home lacked electrical power. In addition, there was no telephone service to residents' rooms on the second floor of the independent living area, and the alarm system, including a strobe horn, a light signaling system, and smoke detectors in each room, was destroyed. The alarm system control panel was located in the attic and melted from the heat.

That night, Mrs. Evans called an electrician, the alarm repair service, and the telephone company. Although the electricity and the phone service would be restored the next day, emergency measures were necessary to allow residents to sleep in the home, especially in rooms at the ends of the hallway where the fire raged.

First, Mrs. Evans arranged for the electrician to connect a cable to provide bright lights in the damaged hallway. Then she established a night watch with the charge nurse and a night watchman who made rounds every ten minutes. This vigil reassured the residents and made them feel comfortable about sleeping in their rooms. The repairman for the alarm system arrived that evening and worked most of the night to install a new system.

The home's staff worked through the night, and after a quick purchase of three industrial vacuums, they removed the water, and with extra mops and rags, tried to dry everything out. Water kept running from the attic for a day and a half. At 3:00 A.M. Mrs. Evans finally had the time to go to a spare room in the home for a few hours sleep. She slept fitfully, continuing to worry about the well-being of the residents.

The Aftermath of the Fire

Damage to the home totalled approximately $500,000. Mrs. Evans and the board of directors tried to turn the near disaster into an opportunity. Since the Christian Home was approaching its centennial, they were considering adding funds to the insurance proceeds to renovate the old building before the upcoming celebration. Six months after the fire, new carpet was installed throughout the building.

After the fire, Mrs. Evans decided to rewrite the fire emergency plan. The major lesson she learned from the fire was that the new plan must be tailored to the institution and to the age and mobility of its residents. It must also be flexible and inclusive enough to apply to any time of the day or night. Ever since the fire, she has wondered what would have happened if it had occurred in the middle of the night when the old and frail residents, all with mobility handicaps, were in bed with their hearing aids on their night stands. She would be sure to include instructions for that contingency in the home's new fire emergency plan.

Case 3

The Dietary Dilemma[*]

Seth B. Goldsmith

Seth B. Goldsmith, Sc.D., J.D., is Professor, Health Policy and Management Program, School of Health Sciences, University of Massachusetts.

> *For a man seldom thinks with more earnestness of anything than he does of his dinner.*
>
> —*Samuel Johnson*

On June 15, just seven months after he had been hired, Ian MacLean, the director of food service at the 200-bed Hebrew Home for the Aged of the Dakotas (HHAD), was asked to meet with Benjamin Jonas, the home's director. For Jonas, who himself had been hired less than a year ago, this meeting was a difficult one because its purpose was to ask MacLean to resign, and if he would not sign a letter of resignation, Jonas was prepared to discharge MacLean.

Jonas began by saying, "Ian, I'm sorry that things have come to this but I think, in light of the problems in food service, it would be best for all of us if you resigned. I warned you last month that this would happen unless the department was straightened out."

MacLean replied, "Resign? Are you kidding? I'm just getting into the rhythm of this place. I know that I've made some mistakes but I think that I am now getting things under control. Are you just angry about my kashruth mistake at the board dinner last week? This kashruth business is a pain and I've worked very hard to get your Jewish dietary laws down, but the whole business about what

---

[*] Fictitious names of both the organization and individuals are used to ensure anonymity.

meats and seafood can't be eaten and the laws against mixing meat and milk aren't second nature to a Scotsman like me."

"Ian, please listen to me carefully," Jonas implored. "The kashruth at the board meeting was clearly a problem. But after being here as long as you have, plus your agreement to study the rules of kashruth, there really is no excuse for ordering the staff to put sour cream on the tables when the dinner is going to be roast beef. You know perfectly well that we never serve dairy and meat at the same meal. By now you should know that all of that cream for the coffee and whipped cream are really non-dairy substitutes. So while I acknowledge that I am annoyed by your putting the sour cream on the table, fortunately Louis [Louis Isaacs, Assistant Administrator] saved the day by checking the dining room out before the board came in and taking the sour cream off the tables. But I think there is something more important. Did you ever wonder why Esther, Max, Julio, and Jill didn't say anything to you since they certainly know better? I'll tell you why. They don't trust or respect you."

"Wait a minute," MacLean interrupted. "I think there is another explanation and that is they were trying to undermine me. I took over a 30-person department that had never had a manager, that was run by the senior cook, and that the state inspector said didn't meet the requirements for proper food handling. You hired me to set up a new tray delivery system and you yourself said I did an outstanding job of that."

This time Jonas interrupted, "Look Ian, you did a great job setting up the tray system, but that is history! I need someone who can manage the department. Last week when we went out to the Jewish Community Center to discuss the senior citizens feeding project you couldn't even justify our bid of $3.37 per meal which is probably considerably under our real costs. I've got a million dollars tied up in your department, one-sixth of my budget, and I need someone who can control what is going on in there."

In a pleading voice Ian MacLean then went on to ask Mr. Jonas for another opportunity to manage the department. Jonas replied that his decision was final; MacLean could resign or be fired. MacLean agreed to resign and Jonas agreed to let him phase out over the next 30 days.

The History of HHAD's Food Service Problems

Ben Jonas's agreement to have MacLean stay on for another 30 days was largely due to his own uncertainty about what to do about food service. When he had accepted the administrator's position ten months earlier, he recognized there was a food service problem but he did not know how serious it was. What was obvious from the outset of his tenure was that the food served at the home lacked variety. The standard joke was, "If it was fish it must be Wednesday." A far more serious problem that emerged shortly after Jonas's arrival was a state inspection report (Exhibit 3-1) that found the food service deficient. The problem was the food handling procedure in which food was delivered in bulk form to the six resident units and then portioned out by the nursing and dietary staff. The state inspectors also evinced concern about a lack of attention to the dietary restriction orders of the physicians.

In response to these problems, in particular the report of the state inspectors, Mr. Jonas asked David Axelrod, president of the home's board, to appoint an ad hoc committee on food service. Because the solution to these problems seemed at the time obvious but expensive, Jonas wanted to make certain that the board was supportive of his first major personnel decision and capital expenditure. After three meetings during a two-month period, the board agreed to fund a new position, director of food services, and allocate $25,000 per year for the director's salary. Secondly, they agreed to allocate $75,000 for a new tray delivery system.

Finding an appropriately qualified food service director turned out to be more problematic than Jonas had anticipated. The response to his blind advertisements in the local and regional papers was disappointing. None of the candidates had experience in managing medium-scale kosher institutions. Almost all the candidates were in assistant manager or shift manager positions at local institutions, particularly schools. Only Ian MacLean stood out as a person who, despite a lack of kosher catering experience, had the experience with systems to implement the tray delivery service. When the HHAD hired MacLean, he was a freelance food service consultant on implementation of new systems. His references all agreed that he had the technical skill to get virtually any size new system up and running on a reasonable schedule. He was called "hardworking," "loyal," and a "nice person." In the two months prior to the tray system installation, MacLean worked 70-80 hours per week and never requested any overtime pay or compensatory time off. He was at the home evenings and virtually every Sunday.

The implementation of the new system was technically flawless. The food arrived at the units in the correct amount, residents received the diets their physicians had ordered, and the food was

Date of Inspection: August 25-26, 19–

1. Sanitation–Stewed prunes and applesauce were stored, uncovered.

2. Disposable glasses and cup liners were used at the breakfast and evening meals.

3. Sufficient numbers of trained personnel were not available to serve and prepare food, e.g., nurses were observed preparing and serving breakfast on the units on two consecutive days of visit. Standard not met.

4. A current diet manual was not readily available at the nursing station. (Floor 1)

5. Sanitation/preparation–Food was observed being served in the hallway, the floor was being washed at the same time. Nurses on all units were observed serving food without hair nets. Standard not met.

6. Menus/nutrition–There was no indication that recommendations by the dietitian regarding iron-rich foods (April and May 198–) for patients with hematocrit levels below normal were brought to the attention of the attending physician. Standard not met.

7. Instructions (place cards) for the serving of special diets were not available at the breakfast meals. A patient on a 2-gram sodium diet received highly salted corned beef; a patient complained that his wife, also a patient, never received her low-sodium diet; nurses, not trained dietary help, serve meals.

8. Of ten patients interviewed, six complained about the food. They said the food was overcooked, that steak was never served, and that the temperatures are better now (implying that the food had been cold).

Exhibit 3-1 Statement of Food Service Deficiencies.

appropriately warm or cool. The system proved to be a boon for the nursing staff who no longer needed to spend over two hours per shift delivering meals, cleaning up, and dealing with the patient discord about portions or flavor.

Reactions to the New Tray System

Despite Jonas's educational effort before the new system was implemented, an effort that included a letter to both the residents and their families about the system, within a week of its installation the complaints about it were overwhelming the administrator. The first problem encountered was a petition from the residents council, an organization of residents that normally confined itself to deliberations about refreshments for various social events. The petition read as follows:

PETITION

Whereas the Residents of the Hebrew Home for the Aged of the Dakotas must consume almost all their meals on the home's premises; and,

Whereas the Residents have selected the home for its kosher food as well as other services; and,

Whereas there has for many years been a tradition of food being served in a family style manner which helps in maintaining a home-like atmosphere at the home;

It is respectfully requested that the former style food service be reinstituted.

Duly made, seconded, and passed by a vote of 14-3 of the residents council, April 1, 19_.

_____

s/ Molly Goldberg, President
Residents Council

    Next, Jonas heard from several board members who, in reaction to complaints from relatives who were residents of the home, brought the problem to Jonas. In response to these complaints, Jonas met with the residents council and sent the following letter to the residents' families:

Hebrew Home for the Aged of the Dakotas
1818 N.W. Chai Street
Fargo, North Dakota

May 1, 19_

Dear Friends:

    As you are aware from my earlier letter on this subject on April 1, 19_ we installed a new food service system at the home. A major overhaul of our food service system was essentially dictated by the state at a recent inspection. Specifically, they found our bulk food delivery system to be unsatisfactory both in terms of sanitary and dietary standards. They were particularly concerned about being unable to properly respond to physician's dietary orders under the bulk system.

After much deliberation, the board and administration selected the Simcha tray system which ensures that your loved ones get their food promptly and properly. So far the system has been in operation for one month and we are pleased with the results.

Change is difficult, but as in this instance, quite necessary. I hope this letter has clarified what is happening with food service. If you would like more information please feel free to contact either me or Louis Isaacs.

Sincerely,

Benjamin B. Jonas
Executive Vice-President

The letter seemed to work. After its mailing the complaints decreased but food service still had problems. The old problems of variety and quality were joined by the new problems of cost and personnel.

Inadequate Food Service Cost Accounting

The need to prepare a bid for the Jewish Community Center's senior citizens feeding project was what brought the cost problem to the fore. The bid required that the home provide detailed data on food costs, preparation costs, transportation costs, and profit margins. As this process was being carried out, it became obvious that cost data for food service were sparse.

The problem of obtaining accurate data was not limited to food service nor was it totally unexpected. It was clear to Jonas from his first day that the home, while having many strengths such as its physical plant and strong community support, had serious weaknesses in management. Problems he identified at the outset included a total lack of a management information system or a purchasing program. Both programs were unsatisfactory and had been under the direction of Assistant Administrator Irwin Brown for many years. As part of his review of costs, Jonas examined the food service cost data sent to the State Commission for Nursing Home Rates. Subsequent discussions with the home's outside accountant and Brown led Jonas to the conclusion that the food service costs were primarily based on trends from data of the previous year. Further, Jonas concluded that the true costs were unknown and that the present accounting systems could simply not account for the costs. For example, each of the resident units had a nourishment station at which were stored tea, coffee, bread, crackers, peanut butter, jelly, juice, and soda. Twice weekly food service restocked these supplies but the expense of this operation was not included in the food service costs.

Finding data about food service was part of Jonas's larger agenda, to develop a state-of-the-art financial management and management information system. To implement this item on his agenda, Jonas proposed at the February 15 board meeting that the board fund a new position for a certified public accountant with both nursing home and computer experience, and fund the purchase of a computer system. The board agreed to this proposal but, because of the home's $500,000 deficit, it asked Jonas to delay the acquisition of the new staff and system until July 1.

Personnel Conflicts

Dealing with the personnel problems was one of Lou Isaacs' responsibilities (the other major one being purchasing). Isaacs, who took over from Brown on January 1, was a recent graduate of the master's program in long-term care administration at the University of Lake Wobegon. His experience in health care management was limited to a one-year administrative residency at the Jewish Home in Lake Wobegon. Before entering the field, he worked for six years as a home contractor in Vermont following two years as a Peace Corps volunteer in Colombia.

Shortly after MacLean began as food service director, the personnel complaints started coming to Isaacs. Within months, at least half of the food service workers had come in at least once to criticize MacLean's management of the department. For example, Max the cook complained, "Ian didn't like the way I cooked the chicken so he complained loudly in the kitchen. It was very embarrassing." Esther complained about his harassing her about productivity: "Lady, why does it take you so long to clean up? You're slower than a mule." Julio also complained about the way MacLean treated him, "I think he's racist. I was on my morning break and meditating and he comes up to me and tells me that we don't allow siestas here." Probably the most crucial problem though was the rumor of a union drive that might attract the food service employees, most of whom, until the beginning of the MacLean regime, were thought to be very loyal to the home.

The Director's Options and Final Decisions

Soliciting MacLean's resignation was difficult for Jonas for both personal and professional reasons. From a personal perspective, he disliked discharging people and he was genuinely appreciative of MacLean's excellent job in implementing the new system. Also, he found MacLean to be charming and engaging. Both Jonas and MacLean were outdoorsmen who shared a passion for skiing and fly fishing, and on a couple of occasions had spent several hours together fishing.

From a professional perspective Jonas had two problems: First, he felt that MacLean was one of his earliest and most visible recruiting decisions and only months later he was discharging this person. After thinking this through, Jonas decided that the embarrassment of admitting a poor decision was outweighed by the damage that was likely to be done if MacLean continued as food service director.

The second professional problem was what to do about the food service department as a whole. Jonas identified several options: (1) allow food service to be managed the way it was before his arrival; that is, the scheduling of employees and departmental management would be done by senior cooks and would be the assistant administrator actively involved in the department (he would essentially function as the parttime food service director); (2) hire a new food service director; or (3) contract out the food services to a contract caterer.

The first option would require the continued active involvement of Louis Isaacs in the management of the department. While Jonas thought that his assistant had a good sense of catering and food service management, it was clear that he was not a food service professional. Additionally, Jonas worried that Isaacs would burn out if he attempted to manage food service as well as carry out his other responsibilities. Finally, complaints from some board members about Isaacs' performance and personality were starting to reach Jonas and he himself was beginning to think that he might need a more seasoned deputy.

After dismissing the first option, Jonas decided to pursue the other two options simultaneously. To develop a pool of candidates for the food service director's position, he contacted the administrators of other nonprofit nursing homes in the region and placed advertisements in local and regional newspapers.

FOOD SERVICE DIRECTOR
Nursing Home & Geriatric Center

Must be experienced in tray systems
and kosher food service. Salary open
based on experience and qualifications.
Send resume to Box 3131
Fargo Gazette

The third option involved using an outside contract caterer. Based on his earlier experience and information he gathered from administrators of other Jewish homes, Jonas invited three firms to make bids on the food service problem. Each company made a two-day survey of the institution and presented Jonas with a formal proposal. All three companies were asked to incorporate the following assumptions into their bids:

1. There will be 72,000 patient days and 216,000 meals per year.

2. The day care program has 24 participants a day, 237 days a year which requires an additional 5,688 meals.

3. There will be congregate meal services (The Jewish Community Center Program) serving 21,000 meals.

4. Free meals are to be served to an estimated 70 persons per day.

5. Subsidized meals are served to approximately 60 staff per day.

6. Food service costs for unit nourishment stations are to be calculated at $.30 per patient day or $21,600 per year.

7. Food service costs for the coffee shop are to be calculated at $5,895.

The problem now faced by Jonas was what to recommend to the board. He received 12 resumes of which five were in the acceptable category (Exhibit 3-2). Three persons were selected for an interview. Additionally, he received three proposals (portions of each appear in Table 3-1). Descriptions of the companies that submitted them are given in Exhibit 3-3. Evaluate the exhibits and decide what you would do if you were Jonas.

Juan Domingo
1314 Green Street
Nashua, New Hampshire

Education

B.S. (1974)	Michigan State University School of Hotel and Restaurant Management E. Lansing, Michigan Major: Institutional Catering
1970-72	Naval School of Hospital Administration Bethesda, Maryland 60 B.S. credits through Abraham Lincoln University

Professional Experience

1955-1967	Hospital Corpsman–attained rank of Chief (E-7) in August, 1966.
1967	Selected for commissioning as Ensign, Medical Service Corps, U.S. Navy
1967-1970	Assistant Personnel Officer Naval Hospital, Adak, Alaska
1974-1978	Food Services Officer Naval Hospital Newport, R.I.
1978-1980	Director of Food Services Naval Medical Center Portsmouth, Virginia
1980-1984	Manager Admiral Sparky's Seafood Emporium Norfolk, Virginia
1984-	Director of Food Services Nashua Hospital Nashua, N.H.

Personal

Divorced
Two children, Juan Jr., 23 and Ilana, 19.
Fluent in Spanish and Portuguese

Exhibit 3-2   Sample resumes of applicants for position of Food Service Director.

William C. Weeks
917 Crescent Street
Lake Wobegon, Minnesota

Employment:
    Since 1985 I have been Manager of the dietary department of the Jewish Nursing Home of Lake Wobegon. The home has 110 residents and a day care center of 10 clients. My department has 11 employees and a budget in excess of $500,000.00. Under my direction labor turnover has been lessened and productivity increased. The number of resident complaints have decreased significantly. I have introduced a variety of innovations including New York Deli night, lox and bagel breakfasts and special holiday meals. Additionally, as part of our activities programs I have taught cooking to the residents and allowed them to come work in our kitchens to prepare their own specialties.
    From 1980-1985 I was assistant director of food services at the Lake Wobegon Medical Center a 200 bed general hospital. In this job I managed a staff of 35 and was involved in the implementation of a tray delivery system.
    From 1975-1980 I was employed by the Royal Catering Company as a marketing representative in The Lake Wobegon and Fargo area. This job involved my working with various institutions that hired the company to provide in-plant catering services. My job involved sales and trouble shooting.
    From 1971-1975 I was an undergraduate student at Johnson and Wales College, Providence, R.I., majoring in Hotel and Restaurant Management. I graduated in 1975 with a B.S. and a G.P.A. of 3.4. At the college I was Vice President of my fraternity, a member of the School choir and active in the Toastmaster's Club.
    I am married to the former Jean Phillips who is a registered nurse, and have two children, Tim, 6 and Becky, 9.

Exhibit 3-2, continued.

S. Gorbaniphar
P.O. Box 514
Fargo, N.D.

Experience:

1987- date	Consultant	Gorbaniphar and Associates Fargo, N.D.
1985-87	Manager	The Lake Wobegon Inn Lake Wobegon, Minn. Salary: $ 29,000 per annum
1983-85	Night Manager	The Fargo Hilton Fargo, N.D. Salary: $ 27,500 per annum
1979-83	Group Manager	The Cyclops Computer Corp. Minneapolis, Minn. Salary: $34,000 per annum.
1974-79	Student	University of Massachusetts School of Engineering Major: Computer Systems Degree: B.S.
1972-74	Student	University of Teheran School of Engineering No degree

Personal:

Married
One child: Avraham, age 4

References:
1. Professor Maxwell Smart, Chairman, Department of Computer Sciences, University of Massachusetts
2. Mr. Adolph Bijou, Owner, Lake Wobegon Inn.
3. Mr. Joseph de Coates, Manager, Fargo Hilton.

Exhibit 3-2, continued.

Mary Anne Davis, R.D.
Dietitian
Fargo Lutheran Hospital
Fargo, North Dakota

Professional Licensure: Registered Dietitian # 01659.

Present Position: (since 1984)	Dietitian at Fargo Lutheran Hospital. Responsibilities include supervision of 3 assistant dietitians and 7 aides. Work closely with Manager of Food services in preparation of therapeutic diets and supervision of staff. Served as acting director of food service in absence of manager.
Previous Position: (1981-84)	Assistant dietitian at Fargo Lutheran. This position involved working with patients and physicians on selecting the most appropriate therapeutic diet. A major part of the job involved monitoring the diets and encouraging patient compliance. Work involved both inpatient and outpatient activities.

EDUCATION

M.P.H. 1981 (Honors)	University of Minnesota School of Public Health Minneapolis, MN Thesis: The cost benefit of therapeutic diets in nursing homes.
B.A. 1979 (Magna Cum Laude)	University of Minnesota School of Home Economics Department of Human Nutrition

Exhibit 3-2, continued.

Gloria Robertson

Job Objective: To secure a senior level food service management position in a progressive and high-quality long-term care facility that will encourage innovative developments and innovative management.

Background:

1. I have a B.A. from Smith College in Northampton, MA. At Smith I majored in Art History and minored in Economics.

2. After graduating from Smith in 1975 I entered a new joint degree program at Columbia University between the School of Business and the School of Human Nutrition receiving both an M.B.A. and an M.S. in Human Nutrition in 1978. In 1969 I received my R.D. certification.

3. From 1978-1981 I was a marketing representative in New England for Pillsbury. This position involved working with wholesale grocers on the introduction of new products. I resigned from this position in order to travel for one year in Europe.

4. From 1982-1985 I worked as Assistant Director of Market Research for the Quest Corporation based in Minneapolis. Quest is a non-profit research center jointly owned by several food manufacturers which does market research on changing eating habits of the population. My particular project involved eating patterns of the institutionalized elderly.

5. Since 1985 I have been a food service consultant for the Chanin Group. The Chanin Group owns 56 nursing homes through the midwest ranging in size from 45 beds to 300 beds. My job involves consulting with contract dietitians and food service managers on improvements in both meeting dietary standards and innovations in systems.

References:
    Professor Mary Wolfe, Smith College, Department of Economics
    Dr. James McGee, President, University of Minnesota, Minneapolis, Minnesota
    Walter Johnsonn, Former Mayor, City of South Minneapolis, Present address: c/o 545 Rio Piedras
        Drive, Ponce, Puerto Rico.
    Ms. Diane White, Vice President for Planning, Rocky Mountain Medical Center, Denver, Colorado.

Exhibit 3-2, continued.

Table 3-1 Summary proposals.

	B. Spoke	Pepper	St. Cloud	Current actual
Food cost	$423,953	$481,316	$417,330	$543,000
Salary	48,000	73,464	104,258	–
Tax/fringe	11,040	20,422	26,065	–
Direct expense	43,200	88,100	63,447	84,000
Non-mgt. salary	329,518	343,816	400,063	546,005
Tax/fringe	75,789	75,639	88,013	120,121
Mgt. fee	36,000	40,000	50,000	–
Subtotal	967,500	1,122,757	1,149,176	1,183,000
Credits				
Cafeteria	20,000	20,000	20,000	20,000
CoffeeShop	13,100	13,100	13,100	13,100
Other	5,000	5,000	5,000	5,000
Total cost	$929,500	$1,084,757	$1,111,076	$1,255,026
Cost/pt. day	$12.91	$15.06	$15.43	$17.43

1. B. Spoke Company

The B. Spoke Company is the largest company devoted to food service management in Jewish nursing homes. Presently, it has 15 homes under contract. In addition to the Jewish homes, B. Spoke has another 75 nonkosher nursing home facilities throughout the country and is a division of a corporation that is the fifth largest industrial caterer.

2. The St. Cloud Company

The St. Cloud Corporation is the largest dietary management firm in the health care field presently having in excess of 400 clients. At present it has a total of four Jewish hospitals and seven Jewish nursing homes under contract and is interested in expanding its nursing home operations in the Fargo area. At present, St. Cloud has the catering contract with Fargo Lutheran Hospital and several other institutions within a hundred-mile radius of Fargo.

3. The Pepper Corporation

The Pepper Corporation is a regional food service firm based in St. Paul, Minnesota. Its primary business is industrial catering but for the past ten years it has been trying to develop a nursing home contract management division. At present it has ten nursing homes under contract, one of which is a 75 bed proprietary facility in Minneapolis that is kosher.

Exhibit 3-3 Overview of companies submitting bids.

Case 4

Team Building at Carson Care: Crisis in Communications*

Henry W. Smorynski

Henry W. Smorynski, Ph.D., is Associate Professor, Department of Health Services Administration, School of Administration and Policy, Sangamon State University.

Sources and Stages of an Impending Crisis

Carson Care Inc. (CCI) is a 250-bed facility, licensed for 60 skilled and 190 intermediate care beds. It is located in a medium-sized midwestern city with a primary service area of 140,000 people. There has been very limited utilization of the facility by families from the surrounding small towns and rural areas. There are 15 other nursing homes within the market area with a combined complement of 1,525 beds. Over the years, CCI has established a reputation for cleanliness and nursing care excellence. In fact, these attributes of the 25-year-old facility were responsible for its purchase, over ten years ago, from a local owner by a national chain. The corporation has a reputation in the industry for innovation in long-term care.

In the past six months, CCI reestablished a 16-bed skilled nursing unit certified by Medicare and began accepting residents needing intravenous and tracheotomy care. It was asked by a local medical school to become a geriatric medical residency training site and to

---

* Fictitious names of both the organization and individuals are used to ensure anonymity.

participate in a joint venture to care for ventilator-dependent and trauma patients requiring more complex and intense levels of treatment. CCI wants to increase its market share of skilled and early hospital discharged (DRG) patients needing extended nursing care services.

The facility's local reputation for nursing care excellence was not matched with a similar reputation for innovation. Two years ago, its management reacted to competitor initiatives by opening a special care unit for patients with Alzheimer's disease. Carson spent most of its efforts positioning itself as one of the top five "good quality" homes in the area. CCI management believed the facility's overall reputation would cement its market share.

Within a few years of purchase, Carson's market position began to erode. The facility experienced administrative chaos. The parent corporation's pride in its administrator development programs and its policy of systematic turnover of administrators for maximal productivity and efficiency was strained by leadership problems at Carson. In a two-year period the facility had three administrators, five nursing directors, and operated with the key positions of assistant director of nursing services and assistant administrator unfilled. The last administrator, whose leadership deficits were linked to the decline in the patient census, nursing care quality, market share, and community image, was fired. Given continuing frustrations over failures to hire an assistant director of nursing services, the administrator created a new position, clinical coordinator, to remove scheduling and staffing burdens from the director of nursing services (DON) (Exhibit 4-1). The DON's added obligations reduced her efficiency and prevented her from working on new, restorative and rehabilitative nursing programs needed by the facility to raise quality and increase census.

Although the corporation and much of Carson's staff placed the blame for the facility's decline on the fired administrator, there were other contributing factors. The previous administrator was a hero to many employees, having successfully waged an anti-union campaign. His open and friendly style and high visibility maintained through visits with all employees on the work units endeared him to the staff. After he left, any new administrator would face an instant credibility problem.

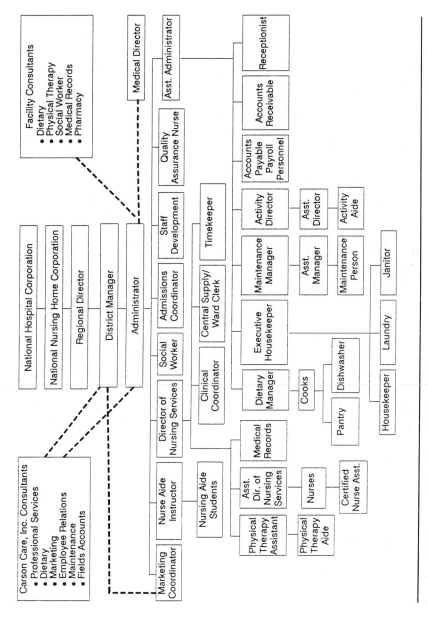

Exhibit 4-1 Carson Care Inc. organization chart.

Externally, Carson's position was challenged by a 175 bed competitor, Salvation Caring Center (SCC), a church-related facility on the affluent west side with a modern physical plant. A strong, church-related admissions base, financial position, and a high private-pay occupancy ratio secured its financial base and positioned it attractively for service diversification and expansion. Retirement homes, continuum of care programs, life-care, and ventilator programs were planned or in developmental stages. SCC was moving rapidly to expand both the upper skilled market (i.e., more complex nursing care as a result of early hospital discharges, ventilator care) and the dependent retirement market (i.e., assisted living).

Other church and proprietary retirement facilities became market factors. Three aggressive home health care agencies were attracting intermediate care patients who could stay in their homes. One was operated by a local teaching hospital which had its own long-term care facility. With the advent of DRGs, this hospital had worked toward vertical integration of all its patient care services.

A third negative factor for CCI was its salary structure for certified nurse assistants (CNAs). Although the parent corporation raised salaries trying to make them competitive, recent surveys indicated that Carson salaries were among the lowest locally for high quality facilities—surpassed only by two poorly regarded municipal facilities (Table 4-1).

The salary structure at Carson could be traced to the shift in ownership. As the acquiring hospital corporation's profits and return on investment deteriorated, significant pressure was applied to the

Table 4-1 Current CNA nursing salary survey.

Facility	Starting salary
Carson Care Inc.	$3.63
Four "quality homes"	$3.84
Municipal facilities	$3.45
Hospitals	$5.00

long-term care division to be more profitable. Concurrently, the state Medicaid program slowed payment schedules and failed to grant increases in basic per diem rates for three years. Medicaid payments were important since 68 percent of Carson's residents were covered through this payment source. The corporation was also frustrated by problems with Medicare intermediaries. Denials of payment had increased over 15 percent in the last six months. Consequently, the nursing home subsidiary was targeted for increased private pay census rates in all facilities over the next year.

Corporate profit pressures and lagging Medicaid payment incentives led to lower nurse staffing ratios. Salary levels fell below those of other service jobs. Long-term care employees could obtain higher starting salaries at local restaurants or cleaning establishments than at Carson Care. CNA turnover rates increased at a time when the facility's nursing leadership was in serious disarray. The previous director of nursing was viewed as arrogant, arbitrary, and unfair by most of the nursing staff. The present DON admitted that the quality of Carson's nurses was lower than those supervised during her hospital experience. She remarked to the staff development coordinator, "I still have no idea of how to motivate them to perform adequately." By April, salary levels and aide turnover were negating nursing care program gains achieved during the previous six months.

Given the deteriorating conditions at Carson, the parent corporation looked for a stabilizing force. It felt conditions required a person with knowledge of the market, and who could rapidly command staff respect. A consultant in CCI's corporate Nursing Section on Professional Services was approached. She had been an assistant director and director of nursing services at Carson when it enjoyed a reputation for nursing excellence. She was appointed as the assistant administrator of the facility and in February was promoted to administrator on June 1 (Table 4-2). Corporate leaders hoped that after stabilizing the facility, she could develop new service lines to attract a higher private-pay census.

The New Administrator Makes Changes

From the outset, the systematic style of the district manager and the aggressive, decisive style of the new administrator clashed. The new administrator did not receive the standard corporate administrator training, extra attention, or support. Rather, the district manager spent a few days at Carson discussing the proper reading, interpreta-

Table 4-2 Chronology of facility events: 198_–198_.

Last Year	Event
February 1	New assistant administrator hired
March 25	New corporate district director named
May 13	Professional social worker hired for first time in facility history
May 21	New staff development coordinator hired
May 23	Administrator fired
June 2	New administrator hired (through promotion of assistant administrator)
July 30	New director of nursing services hired
August 12	New staff development coordinator fills the position left by resignation in July
August 26	Marketing audits program began under marketing coordinator
September 9	New assistant director of nursing services hired
November 5	Census reaches 240
This Year	
February 2	New assistant administrator hired
February 10	Facility begins IV program
February 23	Facility begins internal turnover monitoring in addition to corporation reporting on staff turnover
	Marketing committee created integrating all departments in improving and projecting image
March 24	Department managers meeting sets facility goals and reviews past accomplishments of last six months
June 6-10	Administrator's "chew and counseling" conferences with managers regarding teamwork
June 17	Managers meeting about communication/leadership style of Administrator
June 24	Face-to-face confrontation meeting of whole management team
June 30	New meeting format begins
July 7	All house meeting on communications and the communication audit
July 8-9	Visit of district director and administrator's salary performance review
July 20	Census stands at low 240s

tion, and reporting of corporate financial and budget forms. He explained the corporation's expectations of the facility, identifying clear bottom line measures of administrative performance through census management (i.e., maintenance of more than 240 residents and an increase of 40 percent private-pay residents) and accounts receivable management (i.e., reduction to a 6 percent level by end of this fiscal year). As he left their meeting, the district manager cryptically remarked, "I am only a telephone call away if you ever need my help or advice. Pull it together and good luck."

The new administrator had many strengths and resources to draw upon. A baccalaureate prepared nurse with over five years geriatric nursing experience and a master's degree in health administration (Table 4-3), her management style was to help people grow. She viewed inadequate patient care as the main problem at Carson and

Table 4-3 Management team biographical data.

Position	Time in leadership	Previous adm. exp.	Age	Educ.	Yrs. exp. at Carson	Attend mgr. mtg.
Administrator	13 mos.	3 yrs.	39	M.H.A. B.S.N.	5.5 yrs.	Yes
Assistant administrator	5 mos.	1.5 yrs.	28	M.B.A.	5 mos.	Yes
Director of nursing services	5 mos.	10.5 yrs.	38	Diploma R.N.	9 mos.	Yes
Staff development	11 mos.	None	43	B.S.N.	11 mos.	Yes
Executive housekeeper	18 yrs.	None	44	High school	20 yrs.	Yes
Activity director	6 yrs.	2 yrs.	48	High school	4 yrs.	Yes
Dietary manager	11 mos.	None	44	High school	11 mos.	Yes
Maintenance manager	3 yrs.	None	39	High school	11 yrs.	Yes
Admissions coordinator	9 mos.	None	52	High school	11 yrs.	Yes
Social services designee	10 mos.	None	22	B.S. Soc.Wk.	1 yr.	Yes
Marketing coordinator	13 mos.	None	30	B.S. Hlth. Ed.	4 yrs.	not often
Quality assurance nurse	11 mos.	None	37	L.P.N.	6 yrs.	No

believed that by attacking poor quality on all fronts she could challenge local competitors, retain her best nurses and CNAs, and mold a strong departmental management team. Improvements would be a struggle; the top four managers in the nursing and administration departments had turned over. Nevertheless, she was confident that commitment to a management style that stressed action, performance monitoring, and experimentation would enable CCI to attain corporate goals.

The administrator's instincts told her that an excellent nursing department was impossible with the nursing leadership she inherited. She replaced the existing DON with Carson's best charge nurse and hired a new assistant nursing services director. The district manager criticized this decision; he considered it hasty. He was particularly irritated that he had not been consulted. Within three months the administrator had reconstructed the nursing department's leadership team and was especially pleased with the new assistant director of nursing's leadership potential. In addition, she introduced a full-time quality assurance (QA) position. The QA coordinator reported directly to the administrator and assumed responsibility for the state's inspection of care process, other regulatory procedures, and reporting requirements. The charge nurse appointed to this position was an L.P.N., respected by nursing staff peers for her geriatric clinical knowledge and resident care management style.

Soon after the nursing personnel changes, the administrator had misgivings about the skills and personalities of her new appointees and was particularly concerned about the new director of nursing services. The administrator was confident that the DON would minimize favoritism. However, the DON seemed to make arbitrary professional and management decisions so typical of the fired director. The administrator wondered whether the DON could grow into an effective manager. She had to be content with the fact that she was the best candidate available from a limited pool of applicants. Her familiarity with the facility and commitment to resident care were overriding considerations in the hiring decision.

The administrator had to make rapid census gains. Market competition and mismanagement caused the facility's census to fall to 220 residents last year (Table 4-4). The administrator held several meetings with the social worker, social services designee, and the marketing coordinator about their roles. The administrator had created the marketing coordinator position to launch a new public image campaign; Carson shared the coordinator with another facility in the corporation (75 percent CCI and 25 percent other facility).

The marketing coordinator reviewed the admissions process and was to develop programs and materials to skew the resident mix toward private-pay working with hospital social workers, discharge planners, and other resident referral sources. The social worker was appointed to be the social services designee (the newly appointed

Table 4-4 Average* facility census statistics by quarters and fiscal years.**

Quarter and Year	Total	Private	Medicaid	Medicare	Veterans
Four years ago					
Summer	218.2	60.6	153.1	2.9	1.6
Fall	225.2	65.4	153.0	3.8	3.0
Winter	238.3	74.8	158.5	2.4	2.5
Spring	234.9	65.2	164.8	3.9	1.0
Fiscal year	229.2	66.5	157.4	3.9	1.0
Three years ago					
Summer	240.2	73.5	162.0	3.8	1.6
Fall	245.2	82.4	158.1	2.7	2.0
Winter	233.5	75.4	153.9	2.5	1.6
Spring	224.4	68.3	148.1	4.1	3.9
Fiscal year	236.1	75.0	155.5	3.2	2.3
Two years ago					
Summer	231.7	72.9	154.4	0.5	3.9
Fall	230.0	72.6	155.4	0.3	1.6
Winter	229.3	73.1	153.9	0.0	2.3
Spring	225.5	66.5	155.0	0.0	3.9
Fiscal year	229.2	71.3	154.7	0.2	2.9
One year ago					
Summer last year	232.2	75.5	153.4	0.0	3.3
Fall last year	232.2	74.0	155.3	0.0	2.9
Winter this year	238.4	77.8	157.3	0.0	3.3
Spring this year	238.4	72.7	163.7	0.2	2.0
Fiscal year	233.1	74.2	155.9	0.1	2.9

*These census figures do not match the values reported in the text of the case because they are averages for three months. There was often wide variation in census within a quarter.

**Fiscal year extends from June 1 through May 31. Quarters are June-August (summer); September-November (fall); December-February (winter); and March-May (spring).

admissions coordinator had been social services designee) with primary responsibility for developing and marketing the Alzheimer's unit to prospective families. She also coordinated resident room changes, thereby opening beds for residents drawn to CCI by the admissions coordinator. The goal of these role redefinitions was to increase the visibility and accountability of the admissions coordinator for the facility's census. The administrator firmly believed each individual was capable of stretching to meet these new job requirements.

To support the facility's increasing emphasis on census building, an admissions referral committee was formed whose members included the administrator, director of nursing services, assistant administrator, social services designee, admissions coordinator, and invited participants (e.g., the business office's accounts payable clerk). Meeting frequency grew to three times a week. This increased the admissions coordinator's visibility and allowed for constant monitoring of the admissions process from initial family contact, to floor placement, through resident discharge. Supporting the committee was the new monthly Facility Inquiry Referral Report prepared by the admissions coordinator.

During the first six months under the new leadership, two image and census building strategies were implemented. First, a marketing committee was established to promote the facility as a good place to work, and second, a "Meet and Greet" program was created to provide a positive image through wider participation in community events. The marketing coordinator developed a market audit tool to measure the impact of facility operations on census and the administrator stressed the concepts of customer relations and guest relations.

Committed to management education, the administrator believed that meeting census and patient care goals was impossible without management teamwork. She held inservice training sessions for department managers based on the well-known books, *The One Minute Manager* and *In Search of Excellence*. She enforced the facility's absenteeism policy by reducing the types of acceptable excuses for not working an assigned shift (Tables 4-5 through 4-7). Employees exceeding unexcused absence limits were terminated. She strengthened the daily monitoring of nursing care through new nursing floor rounds assignments. The director of nursing services, administrator, quality assurance nurse, and staff development coordinator (who was also the acting assistant director of nursing services) each monitored the care on one floor during daily rounds and reported their findings to the director of nursing services.

The Facility Improves But Teamwork is Lacking

Having communicated her performance expectations, replaced and retrained key personnel, and developed new reporting/ monitoring systems, the administrator was optimistic about the prospects for quality resident care at CCI. She was confident the census would

Table 4-5 Termination/turnover statistics at Carson Care (in percent of causes given in exit interviews).

Termination cause given	Last year	This year
Voluntary		
Quit with notice	54%	34%
Other	13%	31%
Total voluntary terminations	67%	65%
Involuntary		
Violation of "no call, no show" policy	21%	19%
Inadequate performance through evaluation	9%	5%
Violation of absenteeism policy	3%	11%
Total involuntary termination	33%	35%

begin to rise. In fact, both census and care did respond to the administrator's strategy. Census rose from 220 to 240 in November last year. A marketing audit report this February showed significant quality of care improvements, as did the various reports of the quality assurance nurse.

What bothered the administrator in the winter months was that whereas the quality of care and the census had significantly improved, they had changed little since November. Unfortunately, those levels were acceptable to neither the corporation nor the district manager. Further, some erosion of quality and productivity gains had begun. The accounts receivable position worsened from 7 percent last

Table 4-6 Nursing and overall facility turnover statistics at Carson Care by year and by case.

	2 years ago	Last year	This year
Turnover percentage			
Overall facility turnover percentage	62%	87%	73%
Nursing turnover percentage of facility total	64%	49%	67%
Causes of Turnover in Nursing			
Better pay elsewhere	3%	6%	7%
Inadequate job performance	4%	2%	5%
Absenteeism ("no call-no show" and resignations without notice	59%	42%	32%
Other unspecified causes	34%	50%	56%

December to almost 13 percent by this April (Table 4-8). The turnover in CNA positions increased dramatically. The budget submitted to the corporation was based upon achieving a census of 244 by March and increasing the private-pay base by four residents. The census and private-pay mix remained level from November through June. After initial census rises, the private-pay ratio worsened and patient level of care needs rose.

The administrator began to sense a lack of growth in her department heads as managers. Department head meetings failed to identify problems that were common to all departments. In regard to solving such pervasive problems as excessive floor odors, inadequate preventive maintenance, dietary regimen compliance, and care planning conferences, there was a total absence of information, communication or resource sharing among department heads as a whole

Table 4-7 Short-staffed shifts worked this year by floor, floor type and time period (in percentages* of shifts/total shifts worked).

Nursing Floor	Floor Type	Dec. 15–Feb. 14	Feb. 15–Apr. 15	Apr 15–June 15
First	Light care	28%	43%	56%
Second	Light care	3%	3%	5%
Third	Heavy care	29%	28%	36%
Fourth	Skilled care	14%	11%	11%
Special care unit	Alzheimer care	7%	3%	2%

*Percentages are based on staffing patterns planned and accepted by the corporation and the administration, not merely needs perceptions of nurses or aides. Staffing shortages were recorded if the shift worked for one hour or more with fewer than the schedule number of nurses for the floor at 7:00 A.M. for that day.

Table 4-8 Accounts receivable (AR) percentages.*

Month	Percent AR
December last year	7.0
This year	
January	11.0
February	9.0
March	11.0
April	12.6
May	12.4
June	19.8

*The accounts receivable report is due from the assistant administrator for review and corporate forwarding on the fifth of each month. The June figure was inflated by changes in the state Medicaid payment cycle and did not continue beyond that month.

or even among sub-groups of department heads. Rather, all problem-solving remained within, rather than among, departments. Considerable interdepartmental criticism arose in private administrator and department manager conferences. The administrator concluded that the quality of care and census problems were traceable, at least in part, to the absence of managerial teamwork.

The administrator decided that more aggressive and targeted actions were necessary. She planned to redirect attention to team building and interdepartmental integration. Believing that the key to developing good-willed technical workers into managers is good communications, she increased the frequency and intensity of conferences with department heads. To date, only the maintenance, housekeeping, admissions coordinator, and social services designee team members kept her involved in their non-crisis problem solving process. She delegated specific assignments to the nursing director (specific, mandatory hours for rounds), staff development coordinator (mentoring responsibility for charge nurses), and dietary manager (spot check of food temperatures on dietary carts), and increased their reporting responsibilities.

While she was tightening the communications process, the administrator depended more heavily on the marketing coordinator as an internal auditor. She needed independent and more timely problem identification regarding nursing care and the census. The marketing coordinator was given responsibility for tracking the performance of all departments. Tracking led to action plans involving several departments, with specific time-tables for resolution and reporting. The administrator increased the number of meetings with the marketing coordinator. Many critical reports and action plans emerged from this process in February and March. They generated resentment among senior managers who viewed the marketing coordinator as a spy for the corporation and the district manager.

To verify her sense of the facility's current performance, the administrator also had the marketing coordinator conduct a staff and residents' family satisfaction survey. Survey results showed progress toward the administrator's goals, but they also indicated that more work was needed. Only 36 percent of staff felt that the facility offered excellent patient care. Twenty-eight percent of employees would not recommend the facility as a place to work. Only 50 percent of residents' families rated care given at Carson as excellent while 21 percent felt that the nursing care needs of their relatives and loved ones were not being met. In spite of concerted effort, 35 percent of patients' families were disappointed with facility odor.

These survey results were reinforced the next month when the State Survey Inspection of Care failed to increase the facility's reimbursement and reduced the facility's quality of resident life rating from four to two stars on a six-star scale. Care plan inadequacies, deficiencies in volunteer programming, and inadequate resident activities were cited. The state's decision cost the facility approximately $32,000 (annualized) in revenue.

After the survey, the administrator became much more directive with the DON, staff development coordinator and quality assurance nurse. She insisted that they develop new restorative nursing programs together with inservice training and monitoring. Care was provided but not properly documented, so charge nurse training in charting and care planning was initiated. Care planning conferences had become education/training sessions more than resident needs assessment meetings. Because the time required for the conferences exceeded that which each manager could realistically give, attendance and meeting preparation worsened each week.

The administrator expanded most of her managers' job descriptions, through both the department managers meetings and individual conferences. If a manager did not "take ownership of a problem," another manager was assigned to resolve it. From November through April, more authority and responsibility were given to the quality assurance nurse and the marketing coordinator. The dietary manager, admissions coordinator, activities manager, and housekeeping manager were criticized for poor performance and reporting deficiencies. The DON and the staff development coordinator were criticized for weaknesses in staff scheduling practices, poor floor communications, inadequate nursing rounds, and weak charge nurse supervision.

Staff Rebellion and a Sense of Team Purpose

As the weight of the administrator's second action phase settled on the department managers' shoulders, they bristled, became resentful, abandoned organizational goals, and retreated into their own work. They viewed the administrator's expectations as unrealistic; they felt a desperate need for support in their roles and reduced demands from the administrator.

In April, management team members began to commiserate among themselves. The nursing director and development coordinator rationalized their standards of performance in terms of their acute care backgrounds. Managers of activities, housekeeping, and maintenance formed a support group. As experienced line administrators, they would try to ride out their current leader's initiatives. The marketing coordinator, social services designee, and the admissions coordinator buried themselves in work and reduced their interdepartmental communications. All felt indebted to the administrator for various reasons: first job (Social Services Designee), job beyond one's competence (Admissions Coordinator), and dual-corporate level appointment (Marketing Coordinator). The dietary manager and the new assistant administrator experienced severe adjustment and performance problems. Only the quality assurance nurse supported the administrator's approach.

Department managers believed that the administrator dealt with the symptoms of problems rather than their causes. By early summer, they were behind in completing the administrator's special reports, filing only those required by corporate headquarters. The gap between audited action plans and implemented line actions widened. The managers brought few substantive problem solving issues to the department managers' meeting. They saw too many inconsistencies in the administrator's communications. In a March meeting, she had praised them for facility odor improvements, accounts receivable performance advances, teamwork and census building, while privately criticizing performance in the same areas (Exhibit 4-2). They viewed the administrator's goals list as far too ambitious. By mid-July, 88 percent of the goals had not been realized. In fact, 49 percent of the goal areas were worse than three months earlier.

The administrator feared that management team building was a failure. Problems only reached her at crisis stage. During three department managers meetings in June, the communications bottleneck exploded, partially precipitated by a communications audit prepared by an outside consultant at the request of the administrator.

The audit involved structured, private interviews of employees (Exhibit 4-3) covering interpersonal employee relations, facility leadership, quality of care, productivity improvement, and overall facility coordination issues. Over 115 employees at Carson were interviewed.

Out of frustration with team performance, the administrator decided to "chew" on the individual managers. In the second week of June, before attending a corporate regional managers meeting, she identified a specific problem that each manager was not resolving and criticized their lack of interdepartmental teamwork and communications. As a follow-up, she scheduled individual job expectation meetings. She felt confident that these meetings clarified her positions and that each department manager agreed with her evaluations of their department's problems and the best ways to restore teamwork. The meetings were open, frank, and complete; several managers even made suggestions to improve her own functioning.

While the administrator attended corporate meetings, the managers decided to lunch together. After opening pleasantries, the session evolved into two hours of grievances, feelings, and perceptions about their various "chew and counseling" meetings with the

A. Accomplishments cited by administration over last six months:

- Morale is up
- Census is high
- Improved odor control
- Admitted more Medicare and heavy care patients
- Hired assistant administrator
- Completed refurbishment
- Improved serving time in the kitchen lines
- Department managers are working as a team
- Physical therapy assistant hired
- Special care unit is full
- Improved patient care quality
- Housekeeping improved appearance of third and fourth floors
- Orientation program is working well
- Meet and Greet program inaugurated
- New Central Supply system installed
- Odor committee is active and productive
- Safety committee is more involved, active, and productive
- Marketing committee has been established
- Started Day of Month Program for residents
- Department of the Month Recognition Program is in place
- Admission referral team meetings have been reestablished
- Appointed volunteer coordinator
- Accounts receivable percentages are lower
- Food costs are according to budget
- Weekend administrative coverage has been a success
- *Let's Communicate* newsletter developed

Exhibit 4-2 Accomplishments/goals lists–March meeting.

administrator. The DON was shocked at the intensity of feelings expressed and agreed to serve as group reporter at the next department managers meeting. Several managers made it clear that they would resign if communication and leadership problems were not resolved.

The DON was surprised that the other managers had withheld their true feelings. She enjoyed a good relationship with the admin-

B. Goals for facility and staff for the next six months:

- Establish exercise programs for the fourth floor (Social Services(S.S.)/Physical Therapy(PT)/Activities(Act))
- Hold "family nights" on each floor (Act./S.S.)
- Develop an adopt-a-resident program (Act/Marketing Committee)
- Install a contracture program for residents and arrange for reimbursement (PT/Nursing)
- Develop and expand a volunteer program
- Begin a resident meal-of-the-month function (Activities/Dietary)
- Obtain higher state reimbursement rates through improved documentation of care
- Reduce accounts receivable percentage
- Maintain census level of 240 or higher
- Change resident mix and increase private pay patients by 40 percent
- Lower staff turnover rates
- Improve patient care plans
- Develop small psycho-social groups (i.e., diabetics, patients)
- Complete renovation of laundry area
- Install new showers
- Solve hot water problem
- Conclude refurbishment and make improve facility appearance
- Increase referral sources for resident inquiries
- Prevent "level two" state inspection violations
- Hire occupational therapist and speech consultant
- Prevent fines from the state
- Prevent union activity
- Hire additional management staff
- Celebrate National Nursing Home Week with an open house (Marketing Committee)

Exhibit 4-2, continued.

istrator, but generally followed her own professional and managerial instincts in spite of what the administrator said. She felt indispensable.

The administrator returned, was briefed by the DON, and called a department managers meeting. Those attending were vocal and emotional; the meeting lasted 7 1/2 hours. The marathon session was clearly an effort to re-establish lines of communication. The administrator was upset and shaken by the process, but enlightened by its

Communications and Stress Reduction Discussion Questions

1. Who do you get your best information from to help you perform your daily work?

   a. Is there anyone else that is helpful for information?

2. Why do you trust the individual/s that you believe give you good information?

3. What recent communications related to your job do you remember most? Why?

4. What source (i.e., individual/s) of information do you believe least? Why?

5. What are some major problems affecting your work right now?

   a. Have you discussed these problems with anyone? Has it made any difference?

6. Are there any specific meetings that you believe are very helpful to you in performing your job?

7. How can we improve communication at the facility?

8. How could we reduce your current job stress?

9. If you were in charge of your work unit, what would be the most important change you would make?

Exhibit 4-3 Communications audit

revelations. She restructured the department managers meeting format, and formal agendas became their centerpiece (Exhibit 4-4). Staff members were informed in advance of specific reporting requirements. Managers helped identify the problems for future discussion. Interdepartmental problem solving would be a scheduled part of each meeting. More of the reporting that had been coming directly to the administrator would now be discussed, in preliminary form, with all managers.

June 30, Tuesday, 9 A.M.

Old Business
1. Report on Meet and Greet meeting–admissions coordination
2. Topics for All Staff meeting–Time clocking
3. Marketing coordinator's role (administrator)

New Business
1. Capital budgets Administrator)
2. Garbage disposal (Maintenance)
3. Exit interviews (Staff Development Coordinator)
4. Meeting minutes (Administrator)
5. Health Care Association convention (Administrator)
6. Resident Council meeting (Activities Director)
7. Health Care Association peer review process (Assistant Administrator)
8. Resident privacy (Please read info. before meeting)–(Administrator)

Department Reports
1. Special Care Training--Bring outline for topics and dates (bring 15 copies)
   Report on fourth floor Family Night and special care unit Picnic-(Social Service's Designee)

2. Maintenance monthly checklist (bring 15 copies)– (Maintenance)
3. Range of motion; exercise at meals (Physical Therapy)
4. Employee recognition (staff development coordinator)
5. Kitchen floor (Dietary)
6. Recruitment Problem (Nursing)

Major Problem Report

Odor Buster Group Results from floor testing

Exhibit 4-4 New department managers meeting format.

The Administrator's Lingering Uncertainty

One year after assuming the top administrative post at Carson Care Inc., the administrator hoped that the recent opening of communications and revised format of department managers meetings would foster teamwork and problem resolution. She wondered whether the communications audit had unplugged permanently sluggish communications in the facility. While recuperating from a peptic ulcer attack, she considered additional steps. She knew from experience that teamwork on the nursing floors was hard to achieve and had to be constantly nurtured, and that it was impossible unless it started with the organization's chief executive. Had she finally found the key to energize her team, or were her years of hard work in building quality care at Carson Care all for nought?

Part III

Operations

Introduction

Operational issues presented here include relocation, establishing policies and procedures, developing a client data base, and tracking charges for services delivered. Long-term care administrators show differing levels of direct involvement in daily operational activities of a program or facility. Whether involved directly or indirectly, the administrator sets the tone for operations and approves procedures which result in a level of efficiency and effectiveness.

"Relocation of the Hilltop Care Center" follows the deliberations and activities of the relocation task force which is charged with responsibility for planning the move of a 200-bed nursing facility. In addition to concerns for resident safety, residents' rights, and ongoing provisions of quality of care, the task force also must address family and staff attitudes toward the move.

The case involving the Jackson Nursing Home features meetings of a committee struggling to develop a "Do Not Resuscitate" policy. Immediate concerns for a terminally ill patient complicate and press for the development of operating policies and procedures.

"The Need for a Client Data Base: The Greater Southeast Center for the Aging" is a case set in a vertically integrated health care system that includes a hospital, two nursing homes, an adult day care program, and several community-based long-term care services. Can the organization develop a client data base to determine if the center is meeting its objective of providing a true continuum of care to clients?

The tranquility Health Care Center in "Capturing Lost Charges," loses charges and wastes meals due to breakdowns in normal operating procedures. While problems have been identified, the situation requires new procedures in several areas to eliminate their causes and to allow for increased revenues.

Operations of complex organizations are not static and must change in response to environmental conditions. An administrator's ability to identify needed changes before problems develop, or at least before they become very serious, is critical to the success of the organization.

Case 5

Relocation of the Hilltop Care Center[*]

Donna Lind Infeld and Gary E. Crum

Donna Lind Infeld, Ph.D., is Associate Professor, Department of Health Services Administration, School of Government and Business Administration, The George Washington University.

Gary E. Crum, Ph.D., is Associate Professor, Department of Health Services Administration, School of Government and Business Administration, The George Washington University.

Overview

The Hilltop Care Center was founded and built in 1917. At present 221 residents live in a large building, located in an upper-class residential community of a medium-sized East Coast city. The city had been suffering from a severe shortage of nursing home beds until last year when three new facilities opened. In addition, two other facilities completed renovations which brought previously inactive beds into operation. As a result, the nursing home market became more competitive. In addition, since Hilltop had long been considered one of the best facilities in the area, it always had a long waiting list.

Two years ago, the board of directors of Hilltop Care Center decided to construct a new building. This case describes the process the administration undertook to plan for the move to the new facility.

---

[*] This is a hypothetical case which is based on a real experience of relocating a nursing home.

The Present Center

The Hilltop Care Center is an intermediate care facility with 222 beds of which 12 are in a skilled nursing unit. The center is certified for Medicare and Medicaid. Last year, the facility operated at 99.3 percent occupancy with over 60,000 patient days of care provided and 65 new admissions.

Three wings were added to the original building between 1933 and 1950. The structure is obsolete and in desperate need of repair. The building has five functioning floors, three of which contain resident rooms. Serviced by two very slow elevators, at least one of which regularly fails to function, the building has tall ceilings which give a cold, institutional feeling. Most resident rooms are doubles without baths, and there is a shortage of central bathrooms and shower facilities. Patient care areas are on the second, third, and fourth floors. The second floor contains a large multi-purpose room. The ground floor houses a lobby, dietary, personnel, and several other offices. Administrative offices are on the second and fourth floors.

Most of the current residents have been living at Hilltop for several years. In fact, a review of files showed 11 residents had been there for over 20 years. Some residents' rooms contain personal furniture and other belongings which must be considered in planning the move.

The New Center

Eighteen months ago, a ground breaking ceremony celebrated the construction of a new Hilltop Care Center on the same campus as the current facility. The new building will have many advantages over the old one.. It will have three floors, all above ground, served by four elevators. The overall size will decrease by six beds, resulting in a total of 216 beds, composed of 180 intermediate care and 36 skilled care beds. The configuration of the facility will change from six to five intermediate care units, retaining one skilled care unit. Each unit will have 36 rooms. One unit will be secured for cognitively and behaviorly impaired residents.

All rooms will be private with shared baths between two rooms. Married couples can have adjoining rooms and use one of them as a sitting room. Each resident room will contain a locked area for secure storage of personal possessions. The facility will be very bright, with skylights and atriums providing a feeling of being outdoors. The major common room is a large, unenclosed space on the first floor. Each floor has easy access to an outside, secured courtyard so that residents may enjoy the nice weather whenever they choose. Units have separate nursing stations, designed more like a hospital than a typical nursing home. The floor plan maximizes social interaction among residents by the use of many open common areas.

Administration

As a not-for-profit corporation, the Hilltop Care Center is managed by a voluntary board of directors with 46 members. An executive committee of 12 members is actively involved in decision making for the center. The chief operating officer of the facility is the executive director, Mr. Kurt Phillips, who has been at the Center for five years. Mr. Phillips directs a staff of 225 persons (Exhibit 5-1 and Table 5-1).

Relocation Task Force

The move to the new building was originally scheduled for October of this year. In March, a relocation task force was created to develop a plan to safely and efficiently relocate the residents. The chairperson was the assistant administrator, Mrs. Diamond, who had been employed at Hilltop for less than a year. Other members of the task force, as originally appointed, included the research coordinator (Mrs. Rivers), volunteer coordinator (Miss Carr), director of social services (Miss Borum), director of environmental services (Mr. Miller), and director of nursing (Mrs. Martin). The task force would meet weekly until the move is completed.

The First Task: Research

One of the first activities undertaken by the relocation task force was background research conducted by the part-time research coordinator, Mrs. Rivers. She reviewed the literature on relocation of the elderly and conducted telephone interviews with four nursing homes in the area which had moved in the past ten years. Mrs. Rivers' research revealed aspects of nursing home relocation which the task force and staff carefully considered.

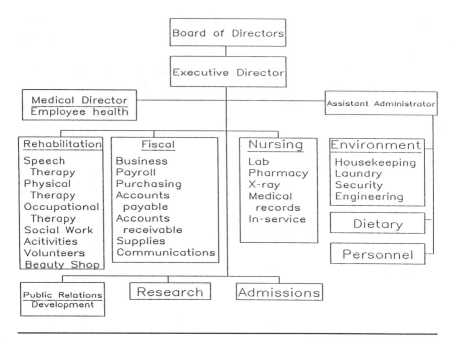

Exhibit 5-1 Hilltop Care Center Organization Chart.

Key Findings. Relocation became a research issue in the 1950s and 1960s when the federal government mandated that nursing facilities improve quality of care, including improvements to the physical plant. Initial research that measured the impact of moves of the elderly revealed increased mortality rates following relocation. Relocation became equated with negative outcomes including increased risk of mortality, and terms such as "transfer trauma" and "relocation shock" became common in the literature on the subject.

Since 1980, when an ongoing debate arose over whether relocation did or did not result in increased mortality rates, researchers have explored ways to reduce the potentially negative consequences. In these studies, the conditions of the move, functional status, health status, and demographic characteristics of residents were considered. Results of the studies revealed that patients who fared best during relocation tended to be female, and were younger, in better physical condition, and had more positive attitudes about the move, compared to the average resident. The report concluded with 11 recommendations for a successful relocation:

Table 5-1 Staffing patterns.

Department	Full-time equivalents
Administration	5.0
Personnel	2.5
Finance	10.5
Development	2.5
Maintenance	4.0
Laundry	6.0
Engineering	3.0
Security	2.5
Dietary	25.0
Housekeeping	15.0
Medical Services	1.5
Rehabilitation	13.0
Nursing Administration	8.0
Nursing	
7:00 A.M.-3:30 P.M.	52.0
3:00 P.M.-11:30 P.M.	36.0
11:00P.M.-7:30 A.M.	31.0
Floating staff	10.0

Note: Each unit includes a nurse with the title of Resident Care Coordinator (RCC) in the morning and a Clinical Specialist in the afternoon and evening. In addition, there is one L.P.N. and four to ten nursing aides depending on the unit and the shift. The skilled unit also has one additional R.N. on each shift. Contract services include pharmacy, radiology, and laboratory.

1. Begin preparation as early as possible.
2. Inform everyone orally and in writing.
3. Maintain steady communication with residents, family and staff.
4. Use a multi-media approach to information.

5. Maximize resident choice and control over the move.

6. Target those residents who are most "at risk" of having difficulty with the move for special preparation efforts.

7. Create an environment supportive of the move by keeping up staff morale about the relocation.

8. To the extent possible, preserve the integrity of the units and make the new physical and social environment similar to the old one.

9. Moving unit by unit in a gradual or phased relocation is preferred to a mass, quick move.

10. Regardless of the timing, the move should be scheduled to provide a minimum amount of disruption to daily routines.

11. Pay careful attention to residents' personal belongings and room furnishings.

Task Force Meetings (April – May)

The first weekly meeting of the relocation task force was held on April 11, at which time the estimated move date was October, so the task force had about six months to make and effect its plans. During the first few months, subcommittees formed to work on the following items identified by the task force.

1. **Building preparation.** Everything to be moved had to be chemically exterminated within three weeks of the move. Primary responsibility for extermination was given to the Director of Environmental Services, Mr. Miller. He was also given the job of ordering transfer materials such as boxes.

2. **Labeling system for boxes and belongings.** The Director of Rehabilitation, Ms. Collins, took responsibility for working on this project.

3. **Unit designations.** The social service and nursing departments worked together to plan resident unit and room designations in the new building. Initial

designations for current residents would be developed in June, with monthly updates.

4. **Staffing issues.** The director of nursing was responsible for staff planning during the move. The facility
would need extra licensed staff so both the old and
new facilities could be operational. Staff would be
asked if they wanted to change shifts or positions
upon moving to the new building.

5. **Communications.** This task was to be handled by the
Research Coordinator, Mrs. Rivers. Starting in May,
the Hilltop Care Center newsletter for residents
would include an article about the move. A publication for families would also regularly begin to contain information about the relocation. The *Bulletin*,
a new newsletter for staff, would report on task force
activities. For example, the first issue of the *Bulletin*
reported on the installation of a suggestion box to
receive input from staff such as questions or concerns
about the move.

Each of the subcommittees developed a chart showing the timing
of necessary steps before the move. The major steps for each activity
are described in Table 5-2.

Initial plans called for a three-person team to move all residents
over a five-day period. Three positions were defined: move coordinator, medical information transfer specialist, and item transfer
specialist. Job descriptions, instructions, and forms for keeping
records of actions during the move were developed for each of these
positions (Exhibits 5-2 through 5-7). These positions were to be filled
by current staff, including some staff volunteers who would earn
overtime pay or compensatory time by working during the move. Because the unit structure would be changed in the new building, the
task force anticipated that units would not be able to be moved
intact.

Task Force Meetings (June)

The Director of Research, Mrs. Rivers, chaired the first meeting
in June because the assistant administrator was unavailable. Mrs.
Rivers reported on her activities regarding communications about
the move. The business office would send a letter to family members

Table 5-2 Relocation preparation schedule.

Activity	Precedent activities	Time frame
Building preparation		
1. Bids for chemical extermination of new building	None	May-June
2. Order materials (boxes, etc.)	None	Apr-July
3. Hire and train new housekeeping employees	None	July
4. Orient maintenance staff to new building	3	Sept
5. Train laundry staff on new equipment	4	Sept
6. Clean new building after turnover	3,4,5	ASAP
7. Clean old building during and after move	None	Ongoing
Labeling System		
1. Identify criteria for choosing system	None	
2. Identify categories of items to be labeled	1	
3. Identify items within each category	1-2	
4. Color code units, offices, etc.	1-3	
5. Determine room numbers in new building	1-4	
6. Identify who is to do labeling	1-3	
7. Control system–Who will keep lists?	None	
8. In-service for labeling system	1-7	
9. Assign labeling jobs	1-4,6-8	
10. Order labels	None	
11. Determine placement of label	None	
12. Perform the labeling	1-9	
13. Check labeling completion	1-10	
Staffing New Facility		
1. Prepare unit fact sheet (resident needs)	None	May
2. Identify criteria for unit assignments	None	May
3. RCCs visit new building	None	May
4. Distribute unit fact sheet to RCCs and clinical supervisors (CSs) on all shifts	1	June
5. Review staffing levels by unit and shift	1	May
6. Prepare questionnaire for unit selection by staff	1-2	May
7. Circulate questionnaire to RCCs and CSs during inservice	3, 5-6	June
8. RCCs and CSs select units	4-7	June
9. Notification of RCC and CS assignments	8	June
10. Circulate unit fact sheet to other staff	9	June
11. Circulate questionnaire to other staff	9	July
12. Selection of units by other staff	8, 10	Aug
13. Notification of unit assignments	12	Aug
Written communication about the move		
1. Install suggestion box	None	May
2. Develop lines of communication	1-2	Ongoing
3. Submit articles for resident newsletter	3	Ongoing
4. Submit articles for *Bulletin*	3	Apr-July Oct
5. Write *News* releases	3	June-Oct
6. Distribute staff questionnaire in paychecks	None	July
7. Mail family questionnaire	None	July-Aug
8. Develop and distribute *Transfer Times*	3,7,8	Aug-Oct

Resident name: _____

Old room number: _____   New room number: _____

All of the medical records, information, and medications for
_____(name) were sealed and readied for transfer at _____(time and date). This
resident is now checked out of Room No. ____ and is to be transferred to Room No. ____.

_____ Medical Information Specialist   _____
Date
_____ Resident Care Coordinator   _____
Date
_____ Transfer Specialist   _____
Date

Exhibit 5-2   Resident transfer form.

Job Description:

1. Will be responsible for collecting, packing, transporting, and delivering all medical information and medications for each resident.

2. Will be responsible for "officially" checking resident out of the old unit and into the new unit by completing the Resident Transfer Form and obtaining the necessary signatures.

3. This person must be a member of The Hilltop Center licensed nursing staff.

Instructions:

1. Obtain a blank Resident Medical Information Checklist for every resident you are assigned to move.

2. A few days prior to the move, locate *all* medical information items that apply to the resident and note them in the first column of the checklist.

3. On moving day, collect all items marked on the checklist using a large envelope for papers and a box for larger items. Make sure that individual items and the box or envelope are labeled.

4. Place the sealed envelope in the box and seal the box. All items should be checked off in the first two columns of the checklist.

5. Complete and sign the first section of the Resident Transfer Form and obtain the signature of the resident care coordinator on the *old* unit.

6. Escort the resident to the *new* unit.

7. Unseal the medical information/supplies box and place in appropriate areas of new unit. Check off on checklist.

8. Complete the bottom section of the Resident Transfer Form and obtain the signature of the Resident Care coordinator on the *new* unit.

Exhibit 5-3   Job description and instructions for medical information transfer specialist.

Resident name: _____ From room:__ To room:__

Medical Information	Location	Located	Packed	Checked-in
Medical record	Nurses station			
Medicines	Medical chart			
Treatment record	Medical chart			
Charting data	Nurses station			
Vital signs record	Nurses station			
I.D. card	Admissions			
Insurance info. card	Nursing office			
Lab orders/results	Nurses station			
Appointments	Bulletin board			
Activity schedule	Nurses station			
Treatment supplies	Supply closet			
Liquor	On unit			

Exhibit 5-4 Resident medical information checklist.

of residents later in June, suggestions were received via the new suggestion box, and a second resident newsletter article was published. A survey asking for suggestions and concerns would be distributed to staff with their paychecks, as requested by the director of nursing.

Nursing Director Martin reported that sample furniture provided by a company bidding for the contract to furnish the new facility was on display in the board room. She asked that Mr. Phillips arrange for a sample room to be set up with various color schemes for residents to view. She also reported that the nursing staff was touring the new facility on a regular basis. Unit assignments of residents were under continual review by the nursing and social work staff. Security during and after the move was a new concern identified by members of the nursing department.

After these brief announcements, discussion turned to a review of how the planning for the move was progressing. Confusion arose

Job Description:

1. Responsible for making sure that everything that is to be moved to the resident's new room is properly packed and labeled.

2. Responsible for keeping, completing, and filing the attached checklist so a complete record of all personal items moved, and their condition prior to the move, is available.

3. Can be anyone affiliated with Hilltop Care Center.

Instructions:

1. Obtain a blank copy of the Resident's Belongings Checklist for every resident you are assigned to move.

2. Prior to moving day, conduct a survey of resident rooms noting all items to be moved. For each item, check the appropriate box in the first column of the checklist. Add to the list as necessary.

3. Check that all items are properly packed and labeled.

4. Check the condition of all items.
   Code: G = good D = damaged

5. The resident is allowed to take one container with him/her during the move. This should fit on his/her lap. Check the fifth column.

6. Immediately before the move, check the room again.

7. Within three days after the move, return to the resident's new room and complete the last two columns of the checklist.

Exhibit 5-5 Job description and instructions for item transfer specialist.

over whether a professional moving company would be hired, which it might be, and whether it would provide guidelines for packing personal belongings. Mrs. Carr asked whether the center was planning to hire a person to coordinate the move. Mrs. Martin asked to involve residents in the packing process and suggested the development of a list of residents who were able to undertake or supervise this task for themselves and for other residents. Miss Borum noted that no one had assumed responsibility for developing a labeling protocol since the director of rehabilitation services had resigned.

Discussion moved to naming the units of the new facility. No one knew if this was a task force responsibility or that of another group so this item was forwarded to the executive staff committee.

Name: _____   From room ____ To room ____

	To be Moved	Packed	Labeled	Pre-Move Cond.	Trans. During Move	Check In	Post-Move Cond.
Furniture Mattress							
Chairs Standard							
Wheelchair							
Desk Chair							
Desk							
Chest of drawers							
T.V. stand							
Other tables							
Other furniture							
Television							
Lamps							
Refrigerator							
Wall hangings							
Clothes from Closets/wardrobes							
Boxes							
Drawers							
Other belongings							
Shoes							
Jewelry							
Nick-knacks							
Books							
Radios							
Blankets							

Exhibit 5-6 Resident's belongings checklist.

To be completed by staff

Resident's name _____   Room number ____

	Action taken-date/initials
1. Missing personal items (please describe)	
2. Structural/environmental concerns (i.e., temperature, plumbing)	
3. Concerns about room fixtures, furniture (including linens, wastebaskets)	
4. Other (please specify)	
Signature of registrant/relationship to resident	Date
Signature of Hilltop Care Center Representative	Date

Exhibit 5-7 Post-move register.

Other questions and concerns raised at this meeting included the need to list furniture to be moved and purchased. Did a list exist, if so, who had it? Also, when should all department managers become involved in the planning process? What should their roles be? Who would move first: administrative staff or residents? Who was planning for the move of staff offices?

In closing the meeting, Mrs. Rivers expressed considerable concern. "We must deal with these questions and the issues they raise quickly so the task force can begin to take concrete steps in preparing for the move."

The second meeting in June opened with Mrs. Diamond asking for a recording secretary for the session. Securing a volunteer, she then asked, "What do we need to talk about today?" One suggestion from the task force was that the group should address the timing of the move of staff offices. After a lengthy debate, the task force decided that most departments could move before residents. In general, executive and management departments (such as administration, business office, public relations, etc.) could be transferred as much as a few weeks before the residents were moved. However, some of the timing decisions were dependent upon a determination of the actual move date. For example, the business office should not move on the first of the month because staff are busy processing payroll. Since many staff members, including members of the relocation task force, had now taken their first tours of the new building, excitement and anticipation about the move was starting to grow.

Task Force Meetings (July)

By the beginning of July, some of the questions raised the previous month were answered. The answers were incorporated into a letter responding to questions raised by the June survey of family members. Their concerns focused on the timing of the move, how the move was to take place, and information about the new facility.

The letter informed residents and friends that the move was planned for the fall, with October 1 as the target date. As described in the letter:

- Before moving residents, inspection of the building and orientation of staff to the new equipment and physical plant would be required.

- The actual move would take place over a weekend (Friday, Saturday, Sunday) to increase the likelihood that family members would be available to assist residents. Considering the comfort and security of residents and the need to coordinate service during the move, the task force agreed that three days would allow for an efficient and smooth transition.

- Since the exact date of the move was unknown, greater specificity was impossible. As much advance notice as possible would be provided to family members.

A moving company would be responsible for moving the center's property, residents' furnishings, and packed boxes; however, the company would not pack. Prior to the move, the social service department would develop a list of each resident's items and each item would be labeled and identified.

All personal possessions (except for one box containing "treasures" and several clothing changes) had to be packed and labeled by moving day. The box of "treasures" would be carried by the resident into the new facility. If the resident or family/friends were unable to pack belongings, then staff or volunteers would pack for them. Packing boxes would be provided by the center.

Each resident would move with the assistance of three people: someone close to the resident to provide emotional support; someone to check furniture, clothing, etc.; and a medical/nursing staff member who would gather all medical items.

The residents' council had been asked to offer input about making room assignment decisions. Units had been designated according to compatible social, emotional, and care needs for residents, but room assignments within appropriate units were not yet made. As soon as the current heat wave was over and the internal construction of the new building was completed, residents and families could tour the new building. A formal dedication ceremony and an "open house" was planned for late November.

Task Force Meetings (August)

At its August meetings, the task force considered the room assignment issue. Nursing and social service staff would assign some residents who needed special supervision to rooms near nursing stations, but a procedure for other residents was needed. The residents' council decided that seniority at the center would be the prime criterion for room selection. The task force had to devise a plan so residents, and/or their family member or representative, could view the rooms and provide input before the final selection was made. To provide flexibility, Mrs. Martin suggested that residents have a choice of two rooms on their assigned unit. In addition, a grievance procedure was needed so residents and family members could express concerns about room allocation decisions.

The task force continued to meet weekly, with a growing feeling of frustration among its members. Mrs. Rivers said, "These task force meetings are less work-oriented and more reporting on what we have *been* doing." Mrs. Diamond, who looked rather discouraged herself, asked, "Why is it so difficult for us to come up with one plan and stick to it? We have accomplished almost nothing and time is running out. What we need to do is to set deadlines for all pending items and then stick to them." Other members of the task force disagreed. One member reminded Mrs. Diamond of how much was planned; she stated "Given that we are all novices at this move, we have really made a lot of progress."

There were some questions about who had the authority to make certain decisions (e.g., naming of the units); there were also questions about hiring or appointing someone to work on this problem full time. Since no new staff was forthcoming, the task force continued to follow the activities outlined in their original plans.

Task Force Meetings (September)

Twelve people, an unusually large turnout, attended the first meeting in September, including Mr. Phillips, the executive director. Attendance had ranged from five to nine people in the past, of which five were reliably present representing nursing, research, volunteers, and maintenance. Some members periodically sent replacements from their departments. Twenty minutes into the meeting, Mr. Phillips noted that no one was taking minutes. Fortunately, it was possible to recreate most of what had transpired.

The first item for discussion was the need to change the makeup of the transfer teams. The original plan called for three-person moving teams. This plan was developed under the assumption that units would not be moved intact, therefore it would not be possible to move charts and medications by unit. However, two things changed. After preliminary planning by the group working on unit designations, it became clear that most units would be moving *almost* intact. Also, it was determined that if each resident needed a three-person team, there would not be enough staff to provide the needed assistance.

It was also decided that housekeeping staff could move the boxes containing residents' personal items after the resident moved, as long as they were transferred the same day. A box was too clumsy for a person's lap, so a plastic carrying bag which would hold the medical chart and medications was substituted. Now, only one person would be needed to accompany the resident during the move. A family member or volunteer could wait at the new room to help the resident get settled.

Mr. Phillips then brought the group up to date on the expected time frame for the move:

- The contractor might turn the building ownership over as soon as October 1, but October 15–21 seemed to be more realistic dates.

- After "turnover," staff could have access to the new center to conduct training and orientation sessions.

- New furniture should arrive between December 1 and 10, but old furniture could be used temporarily.

- A dedication event was planned for December 19.

- The state inspection survey could take place any time after December 23.

- Facility licensure would follow inspection by three weeks or more.

Mr. Phillips knew of a local facility which had to wait six months for some structural changes demanded through the inspection process before its move could take place. Conservatively, the most likely date for the move was projected for the second or third week in February. While the group seemed somewhat disappointed at the delay, it was not unexpected.

Mrs. Rivers called the second task force meeting of September to order. The meeting was attended by the volunteer coordinator, a representative from nursing, and the director of environmental services. The task force decided on an agenda for reviewing the plan for the day of the move as discussed and revised at several previous meetings. The task force agreed that the following steps of the plan were firm:

1. The move would take place over a period of three days, two of which would be weekend days so family members could assist. (Forty-five family members indicated availability to assist with the move. It was still necessary to calculate how many additional staff and volunteers would be needed on moving day.)

2. Thirty-six residents would move in the morning and 36 in the afternoon of each day. There would be enough new beds in place for the first group to move, but after that, existing beds would have to be cleaned and transported before further residents could be transferred. There would be three housekeeping crews working. One would clean beds, another would move them, and a third would move personal belongings.

3. The kitchen would open early so that the move could begin at 8:00 A.M. Residents would be awakened at 4:00 A.M. so they could be dressed and prepared for the move. Breakfast would begin a 7:00 A.M. so the licensure requirement regarding a maximum of 14 hours between meals would not be violated. Residents would then move to the multi-purpose room on the second floor where staff would serve a pancake breakfast (brunch/lunch for subsequent groups). Since residents would be very anxious during the wait, the activities department would provide entertainment.

4. A ramp and canopy would provide protection at the point where the two buildings were closest.

5. The moving company would transfer all furniture, however, neither bids nor a contract for this job had yet been solicited.

6. All residents would move via wheelchairs unless a stretcher was required. An ambulance could be used if needed but would not be on call throughout the move.

7. Security guards would be located at key positions to prevent theft of belongings.

8. Designated key staff members would be equipped with walkie-talkies in both buildings.

New ideas and suggestions were also introduced at this meeting. For example, it was decided that residents should move in pairs to prevent overcrowding the elevators and so residents would have company during the stress of the move. It was also suggested that a command center be established where a designated coordinator would monitor the progress of the move and designate other staff members to resolve problems as they develop.

It was agreed that there should be some temporary nurses available to ensure that medications would be administered properly. Consequently, it was also decided that all residents should wear name bands on their wrists during the move.

A simulation of the move was recommended to determine how much time it would take to manipulate someone in a wheelchair down the slow elevator of the old building. It was also stated that there was still need for a labeling system and purchase of labels.

Towards the close of the meeting, the executive director, Mr. Phillips, excitedly addressed the task force concerning some major new developments in the survey and certification process required for the new center. He explained that instead of doing a full survey, the state agency decided that it would only do a "walk-through" of one unit after which a 90-day provisional license to operate could be granted. In this way, a full survey would be delayed until three months after the move. This prompted a new time schedule. The contractor would turn the building over on or about October 4 (three weeks from the date of the meeting). As soon as one unit could be ready with new beds (even if the other new furniture had not arrived), the surveyors could conduct their walk-through. A good estimate for the date of the move would be early November—three months earlier than had been discussed just one week before and only two months from the meeting date!

Given this new time frame, a few issues became critical. The nursing service department had to decide when to stop admissions so there would be sufficient beds in the new facility at the time of transfer. Room assignments had to be finalized. Many details remained unresolved and task force members knew that much had to be done in a short time.

Conclusion

There are numerous issues to consider in analyzing this case. Five topical areas to examine are planning, task force structure and process, communications, impact on staff, and impact on residents and families. Planning for a move of over 200 disabled nursing home residents, their belongings, and staff would be a complex process in the best of circumstances. With only two months to go, effective planning and decision making was critical.

Case 6

Do Not Resuscitate!: A View of a Nursing Home Ethics Committee*

Gary E. Crum and Jared I. Falek

Gary E. Crum, Ph.D. is Associate Professor, Health services Administration, School of Government and Business Administration, The George Washington University.

Jared I. Falek, Ph.D., is Executive Director, Washington Home and Hospice, Washington, D.C.

Octogenarian Mary Lou Dawkins Smythe left the Jackson Nursing Home annual christmas carol sing-along, pushed in her wheelchair by a nurse's aide. They went up the elevator to the second floor, where Mrs. Smythe had the only private room and bath in the home. As they got to her room, she began to complain of dizziness and nausea. The aide hurried Mrs. Smythe into her bed, so she could get a basin. As the aide lifted Mrs. Smythe from the wheelchair to the bed, Mrs. Smythe suffered a massive stroke and went into a deep coma. Mrs. Smythe's physician, the nursing home's medical director, was called immediately. When Dr. Keithson arrived, he saw at once that the situation was critical.

---

* This case is based on a real patient care episode, but the names in the case have been changed and the medical care and organizational responses have been fabricated by the authors in order to address several typical problems documented in the literature on ethics committees.

105

Overview

Jackson Nursing Home, built in 1970, is licensed for 60 intermediate care and 20 skilled care beds. The home is located in Jackson, a small town about 60 miles from the nearest hospital, Springfield City Memorial. Jackson had fallen on hard times since the only large employer, the shoe factory, moved to Springfield City three years ago. The home's occupancy rate dropped from 95 percent to 75 percent since that time.

The home has had the same administrator, Mr. Ralph Baker, for over 20 years and recently hired a young assistant administrator, Jane Adams. The home's board of directors includes five local businessmen who meet annually for about 30 minutes. Mr. Baker openly discourages the board from meeting more often. When it does meet, he gives the members simple decisions to rubber stamp—issues that are seldom at the top of Mr. Baker's own list of priorities. Mr. Baker feels that a good board should "be neither seen nor heard."

It was the day before Christmas and the new assistant administrator, Ms. Adams, was really worried. At 1:30 P.M. she was supposed to chair the first meeting of the Ethics Committee for Jackson Nursing Home. The committee was approved by the board of directors the day before Mr. Baker hired Jane, less than six weeks ago. The board had simply endorsed Mr. Baker's proposal that the administrative staff create the committee, that it meet as needed, and that it be chaired by the home's administrator, Mr. Ralph Baker, or his designee. Jane, as the staff person with responsibility for risk management, had been so designated by Mr. Baker.

When Jane learned there was a problem between Mrs. Smythe's family and the home's medical director, she was sorry she had not previously ironed out some policies and procedures for the committee. Unfortunately, the home's Expected Death and Do Not Resuscitate Orders policy did not provide adequate guidance (Exhibit 6-1). Earlier that morning she had phoned Dr. Keithson, Ms. Landers (the home's nursing director), and Rev. Finnerty (the home's chaplin), asking them to meet her in the conference room. As she entered the conference room, she noted that all three had already arrived.

SUBJECT: _____   POLICY NO: _____

Expected Death and Do Not Resuscitate Orders

When death is expected and unavoidable or when vigorous resuscitation efforts have been declined in advance, do not call the rescue squad; rely instead on the following steps:

1. The attending physician writes an order, "Do not resuscitate," on the physician order sheet.

2. On the progress note, the physician notes that this decision has been discussed, understood, and agreed upon by the resident and/or responsible party.

3. Nurse administrators will assure that all nursing personnel on all shifts are aware of the order by transcribing the order on the nursing card.

4. The order is reviewed and re-signed every 30 days with the monthly orders.

5. An order against resuscitation may be taken over the telephone by a registered nurse while another employee listens to verify the order. The recording nurse should document the physician's rationale, and that the family has been notified. The physician must countersign the order within 48 hours.

Unwitnessed Death

The effort to restart a heart in a resident whose cardiac arrest was not witnessed is virtually certain to fail. A nurse need not initiate resuscitation procedures when a resident is found dead and is likely to have been without a pulse for more than a few minutes.

Exhibit 6-1 Jackson Nursing Home Expected Death and Do Not Resuscitate orders.

Jane: Thank you all for coming on such short notice. It is important that we deal with the problem of Mrs. Smythe as soon as possible.

Dr. Keithson: Luckily you caught me before I left on vacation— though I cannot stay long if I am to catch the limo to the airport. However, I could have had my partner, Dr. Jones, fill in for me, if that is necessary.

Jane: I am not sure he could have filled in for you on this one since you have been the one in direct contact with the patient's family over the last 24 hours.

Ms. Landers: Yes, Doctor, it is important that you are here.

Dr. Keithson: Well, anyway, here I am. What are we supposed to do at this meeting?

Jane: We need to deal with the problem of whether or not we place Mrs. Smythe under a "no code" order. As you all are aware, the family and Dr. Keithson have been in some disagreement about this.

Dr. Keithson: I would rather put it this way: one family member in particular, the older brother of the patient, feels the patient should not be resuscitated if she goes into cardiac arrest, which is quite possible given her history of heart problems and her current coma. I agree with the older brother in this situation. However, the younger brother of the patient believes that she might recover and should have even the most heroic measures taken to keep her alive. I have explained to him that in my opinion, the patient has less than a four percent chance of surviving this massive stroke and regaining consciousness. He is unwilling to listen to reason.

Rev. Finnerty: In cases such as this, reason is not always easy to define.

Dr. Keithson: I feel that the "no code" order should be written, and that oral direction should be given to the nurse in charge of Mrs. Smythe. Unfortunately, she felt that this issue should be kicked upstairs, and therefore that is apparently why we are here.

Ms. Landers: I asked for this meeting because the nurse felt that the "do not resuscitate" order was inappropriate. She had personally talked to Mrs. Smythe's younger brother and he had said that Mrs. Smythe would have wanted to be kept alive. She also felt that if Dr. Keithson wanted to write a "no code" that he should do it in writing, not over the phone.

Dr. Keithson: As I explained over the phone to the nurse, it is indeed ideal to do it in writing so it can become part of the patient's medical record, but it is not always possible. I was planning to go on vacation and it could wait a week. Of course, now that this meeting has been called, I can do it in writing before I leave today. I just felt that it could wait.

Ms. Landers: A week is too long.

Rev. Finnerty: Ms. Landers, you say the younger brother felt that the patient would have wanted to be kept alive under these circumstances?

Ms. Landers: That is what my nurse tells me.

Rev. Finnerty: That is an important fact, and one that we should pursue. Can we verify that?

Jane: I guess we could ask him to meet with us.

Dr. Keithson: I am opposed to bringing in both brothers, but especially to bringing in just one of them. The family members are as old as Mrs. Smythe, and are not particularly educated. They have little understanding of the medical and the ethical nuances in these situations. We, around this table should perhaps be involved, but we should keep it among ourselves.

Rev. Finnerty: I agree with Dr. Keithson that we should not have only one family member in. I think we should have both.

Jane: I have not met the older brother. He only has been here about two times in the last year. The younger brother has been the main one with whom we have been in contact. There are no other family members alive.

Dr. Keithson: The older brother lives in Springfield, about sixty miles away. It was a toll call when I talked to him about his sister's stroke.

Rev. Finnerty: And he said that he agreed to the "no code"?

Dr. Keithson: Yes, he was sorry to hear about her stroke, and he said that he disagreed about his younger brother's decision not to permit a "no code."

Ms. Landers: You told him about the younger brother's decision?

Dr. Keithson: Yes, his younger brother had not felt able to call him since he, the younger brother, was quite upset about their sister's condition. I think once he gets over the shock he will be glad that we decided to go along with the older brother's decision in favor of "no code," assuming that we do.

Ms. Landers: Jane, what is the authority of this committee to make the decision in this matter. Are we just advisory or do we have some legal standing?

Jane: We do not have a policy on that yet, but I would say that we are advisory and also still have some legal standing. Our decision will become part of Mrs. Smythe's record.

Dr. Keithson: If this is just an advisory committee, I must say that I am relieved. I would like to hear your opinions on this matter, but I disagree with the idea that the decision of this committee should become part of the patient's record. If the committee happens to advise contrary to the physician's decision, it will only cause problems for the patient, the doctor, and most of all for the home itself. We want to avoid law suits, don't we, Jane?

Jane: I can certainly say yes to that question.

Dr. Keithson: Of course. Therefore, I propose the following: that I go up to the nurse's station outside of Mrs. Smythe's room and write the "no code" order. The rest of you can draw up a recommendation and present it to me when I return from vacation. My cousin, Dr. Jones, will be covering for me while I am gone. He will see that Mrs. Smythe is comfortable until the end comes. That should pretty well take care of matters.

Jane: What if she is one of the four percent who survive?

Dr. Keithson: Well, that is what we are discussing here. If we write a "no code" order, she will have almost zero chance of surviving. Let me be blunt: no matter how much we try to help her, what we will be doing is only prolonging her death. She is arthritic, has hardening of the arteries, has had a massive stroke, is too sick to move over the snowy roads to the hospital, and has a painful chronic gallbladder problem. This patient should not be resuscitated, period. Let's let her die with dignity.

Jane: No one wants to cause the patient more problems, but we also don't want to sweep her under the rug. About the advisory nature of this committee's decisions, in my opinion it would entail more than a confidential note to the physician involved. The committee's advice would indeed have to be part of the patient's record.

Dr. Keithson: I am very upset to hear you say that. The physician is responsible for the patient, and I have made my decision in accord with the wishes of the patient's family. I see no further reason to discuss it. I am leaving to write the "no code" order, and if it has been changed before I return, I will take the matter to the home's board of directors. I advise you not to try to practice medicine in my absence.

After Dr. Keithson stormed out of the room, the remaining Committee members decided to take a 15-minute break. Jane hurried to her office and called the home's attorney, Penelope Richards. Penelope said that she would come over immediately and meet with the Committee.

Jane: Let's reconvene. All of you have probably met Ms. Richards, the home's attorney. I have asked her to sit in on the remainder of the meeting and provide some guidance. Ms. Richards?

Ms. Richards: I am glad that I was available on short notice. I feel that this committee should have legal input each time it meets. Given Jane's briefing, it appears to me you need to ascertain the true feelings of the two brothers as soon as possible. Of particular importance is the alleged statement by the younger brother that the patient would not have wanted a "no code" order. It would also be helpful to have another medical opinion on Mrs. Smythe's prognosis.

Ms. Landers: Penelope, do you think we should make the two brothers members of this committee?

Ms. Richards: That is not necessary, but I do feel that you are putting the home at risk unless you get more than hearsay regarding the two brothers' positions. These matters are usually handled by the patient's family and the physician, but since the matter has been taken to the committee by the nursing staff, the committee probably must take some official position. This is particularly a risky situation, legally, because the home, to my knowledge, has never established a facility-wide policy on "no code" orders. Whether the committee has the authority to overturn the physician in charge of the patient, or if it only has an advisory role, its ruling could have important legal consequences for the home. In effect, it sets precedent for a facility-wide "no code" policy. Even an advisory role gives the committee quite a bit of authority and responsibility by placing a greater responsibility on the physician to get his or her legal and medical situation in order in case there is a suit.

Jane: Well, would someone like to make a motion?

Rev. Finnerty: I move that we make the two brothers members of this committee for this particular case.

Ms. Richards: Can I second that motion?

Jane: I guess so. The board did not set the membership, and we have not dealt with membership through an administrative action.

Ms. Richards: If I am a member of this committee, then I as your lawyer will have to express surprise and concern. The answer to my question, I hoped, would have been no. The answer you give is one that suggests that this committee has no clear mission, membership, or procedures for acting. This worries me. We need to organize ourselves better before we try to take up such difficult issues. For example, if the committee feels it has the power to overturn the physician's orders, it probably should have at least one physician, preferably two, as part of its membership.

Jane: I think that is a good idea for the future, but right now we have a life and death situation on our hands. We can't take the time. I suggest that we approve Rev. Finnerty's motion and also ask that Dr. Jones serve on the committee while Dr. Keithson is on vacation. Does everyone agree?

Ms. Landers: I would like to make a substitute motion: that we get in touch with the two brothers right now and ask them for their input. Meanwhile, we should make the deliberations of the committee advisory only, and the voting membership will be the people in this room and also Dr. Keithson. Even in his absence I believe, we can assume he is in favor of the "no code" order.

Ms. Richards: This approach to try and make things legal is not appropriate. I would like to recommend that the motion be for the committee to disband until some minimal policies and procedures are set up. It can be done in a day, if the board has truly delegated this authority to the administration.

Jane: I have a memo from Mr. Baker delegating the drafting of those policies to me. Let me draw up some policies and procedures this afternoon. We can meet at 4:00 P.M. and take some action. I will also see if the two brothers can join us, either as members of the committee or just to give testimony. It may be less than ideal, but it will at least mean that we have some internal policies to act upon before we take a position on Mrs. Smythe.

As the committee broke up, Ms. Landers approached Jane saying she hoped the committee membership would include a neutral physician in addition to the attending physician, to give a second opinion when needed. Jane said she would think about this, but was not sure that it was really needed. Ms. Landers said that getting in touch with the younger brother would be easy since he was upstairs in his sister's room right now. He had been at the home all night. Ms. Landers said she would make sure he stayed for the 4:00 P.M. meeting, but that she felt he might be too distraught to be of much help.

Jane rushed back to the administrative suite and looked for Mr. Baker. His secretary said that he had left for the afternoon, but could be reached at home where he was wrapping Christmas presents for his children.

Jane went into her office and closed the door. She called the older brother, Thurston Dawkins, and he reluctantly agreed to come. One hour later, when she called Mr. Baker, she had a short draft to read him regarding the committee's policies and procedures. She decided not to mention Dr. Keithson's threat so as not to upset Mr. Baker. It would appear as if she could not handle things if she gave him the full details about what the meeting had been like.

Mr. Baker said the draft sounded fine and gave his approval. He told Jane to go ahead and sign his name to the final version. He added that Mrs. Smythe, via her annual gift of $25,000 to Jackson Nursing Home, was the single greatest source of income to the home when it was in the red. He said he hoped she would do all she could to see that the "no code" order was at least postponed until the end of the calendar year.

Jane quickly had the draft typed in final version, making only one small change concerning the percentage required for a quorum, signed Mr. Baker's name, and made some copies. She looked at the clock; it was 4:00 P.M. Hurrying to the conference room, she entered and noticed the two brothers sitting silently in chairs down the hall from the conference room.

Jane: Here are the official policies and procedures for the home, as approved by Mr. Baker, and in accord with the directives given Mr. Baker by the board at its last meeting. Of course since this is the first time you have seen them, I will read them for you.

Ethics Committee Policies and Procedures
Jackson Nursing Home

Mission: To oversee the home's activities in the field of ethics.

Membership: The permanent members of the committee are: Mr. Baker or his designee, Ms. Richards, Ms. Landers, Dr. Keithson, and Rev. Finnerty. Other persons can be temporarily added as voting members by a majority vote of the other members that are present.

Meetings: Meetings can be called at the request of any member of the committee or at the request of a patient or a patient's family member. Meetings will take place within 24 hours of the request. A quorum will be at least 50 percent of the permanent members. Detailed minutes of each meeting will be kept.

Authority: The committee will only have advisory authority. In the event that it reaches a conclusion that is opposed by a family member, a care-giver, or by others involved in the case being reviewed, the committee will seek a statement for the record from those in opposition to the committee's position/advice.

In addition to dealing with specific patient cases, the committee will develop educational materials for the home's staff on ethical issues in long-term care.

Ms. Richards: This is not very detailed, but it answers the key questions facing us about as well as can be expected on such short notice. I think we can clean it up and add some more clauses to it at our next meeting.

Rev. Finnerty: Considering how little time we have, it seems adequate to permit us to reach some conclusion on Mrs. Smythe, I believe.

Ms. Landers: I would like to move that we add a physician temporarily to our committee, but I doubt that we can get one on such short notice. I asked Dr. Phillips if he would come to this meeting and serve as a member of the Committee—I happened to know him from the singles group at our church—but he refused because he felt his being an obstetrician made him an unlikely candidate.

Ms. Richards: Since the factory left, there aren't really any physicians nearby except Dr. Phillips and Dr. Katzman, the internist. Maybe we can get Dr. Katzman?

Jane: He is on vacation. If Dr. Phillips isn't willing, then that leaves Dr. Jones, Dr. Keithson's partner, as the only likely source of a second opinion. That is probably not ideal.

Ms. Richards: Let's just listen to the two brothers and then decide what we need before we can make a decision.

Jane: Would you mind showing them in, Ms. Landers?

Ms. Landers: No, but which one should we bring in first?

Jane: Let's bring in the younger brother first. He is so upset about his sister's condition that I suspect he would like to get his meeting with us over as soon as possible.

Ms. Landers left and soon returned with the younger brother, Mr. Y. Leon Dawkins.

Jane: Mr. Dawkins, we are sorry to have to bother you at this difficult time, but we are reviewing your sister's case and are seeking to reach a recommendation about whether she should be resuscitated—whether she should be kept alive—if she has a heart attack.

As you know, it is not likely that she will live long even if she is kept alive by heroic measures. We are anxious not to prolong her discomfort unnecessarily. I understand that Dr. Keithson has talked with you about this?

Leon Dawkins: Yes.

Jane: What do you think should be done?

Leon Dawkins: I want my sister kept alive.

Jane: But you realize that we cannot guarantee that.

Leon Dawkins: I mean I want you to try to keep her alive.

Jane: Are you aware that your brother and your sister's physician both feel that she should not receive heroic measures if she has a heart attack. That they feel she should be permitted to die rather than be kept alive unnecessarily?

Leon Dawkins: What do you mean "unnecessarily"?

Rev. Finnerty: Permit me, Jane. . .Mr. Dawkins, none of us wants to see your sister die, but at times it becomes necessary to stop trying to keep people alive with extraordinary—heroic—measures. The likelihood that your sister will return from her coma is very slight even with this extraordinary care. Do you want to put her through that hardship and expense?

Leon Dawkins: Since her husband died, the estate pays all her bills, and she isn't facing any hardship. She's as peaceful as can be, my poor Mary Lou.

Ms. Landers: Did your sister ever say whether or not she would like to be let go if she reached a place like this?

Leon Dawkins: Well, she refused to sign that living will thing that Dr. Keithson gave her last year. She told me that she thought the whole idea was evil. She said life was too precious to ever sign away.

Ms. Landers: The committee is probably aware that Dr. Keithson often gives the patient or the family a copy of the living will that was approved by the state legislature three years ago.

Ms. Richards: Yes, I have encouraged this, though I prefer the durable power of attorney to the living will, myself.

Leon Dawkins: All I know is that she is alive, and I don't want to see her dead. If she was here, I know she would say the same thing. That's all I have to say, I'm going back to her room now.

Jane: Thank you for coming to speak with us, please be assured that we only want to help.

As Mr. Dawkins left the room, Ms. Landers left with him and asked the older brother, Thurston, to come into the conference room.

Jane: Mr. Thurston Dawkins, we are members of the nursing home's Ethics Committee and we are looking into your sister's situation. We want to see if there is anything that we can do to help.

Thurston Dawkins: I have talked the whole thing over with Dr. Keithson, in fact I spoke to him last only just before I drove over here on the short notice you gave me. I had a rough time getting here in my old pickup in the snow. I suppose you would have gone on without me if I was late.

Jane: No, we need to speak with you before we can decide what to do about your sister's case. We would have waited.

Thurston Dawkins: In that case maybe you can give people more time in the future. . .especially on a holiday. The traffic is stiff and the gas is extra expensive.

Jane: Mr. Dawkins, can you tell us what you feel is the best thing for your sister? Do you feel we should stop trying heroic measures to keep her alive?

Thurston Dawkins: I think you are only prolonging her death. She is real sick and she should be allowed to die with dignity.

Jane: Do you know anything that might help us to decide what your sister might say if she was here today?

Thurston Dawkins: No, except that I imagine she would agree with me and her doctor. If she could only see herself now, she wouldn't want to be kept alive. She was always spunky when she was well, and may have told Leon some stuff that I would expect she would not say now. She would want to die.

Jane: Thank you, Mr. Dawkins.

As the elder Mr. Dawkins left, Jane addressed the committee. Well, is there anyone else we should talk to, or would someone like to make a motion about Mrs. Smythe's "no code" order?

Case 7

The Need for a Client Data Base: The Greater Southeast Center for the Aging*

Philip N. Reeves

Philip N. Reeves, DBA, FACHE, is Professor of Health Services Administration, School of Government and Business Administration, The George Washington University.

The Greater Southeast Community Center for the Aging (CFA) grew rapidly from a small senior activities program located in vacant hospital space to a dispersed, multi-facility, diversified service system. As it approached its tenth anniversary, senior management became increasingly concerned about whether the organization was achieving its major goal of developing a comprehensive continuum of care for the elderly. A positive answer to management's question would mean that clients were being provided appropriate services within an integrated services system. On the other hand, clients might simply be receiving services from several components on an ad hoc basis. If that were the case, management would either have to devise new methods to achieve service integration or modify its aspirations.

---

* This case describes a situation that occurred within a very complex organization existing in a dynamic environment. Although all of the facts presented are essentially correct, it has been necessary to simplify many of the issues which do not bear directly on the solution to the case so that the description would be of reasonable length.

When management confronted this strategic issue, it became apparent that data needed to evaluate the center's achievement of this aspect of its mission were not available. Management decided to correct this deficiency by establishing a centralized client data base. In order to make the undertaking feasible, it was decided that the data base should support strategic and operational decision making. Since CFA also had an active research component, the data base should meet those needs as well.

General Environment

CFA is located in Southeast Washington, District of Columbia (D.C.) (Exhibit 7-1). This area is variously designated as Anacostia and East of the River because the Anacostia River is its major boundary feature and separates the area from the remainder of the city. A patient origin study confirmed that this region, comprised of three ZIP code areas, was the primary service area for CFA's major programs. Three adjacent ZIP code areas in Prince Georges County, Maryland were regarded as a secondary service area. They provided a substantial proportion of the effective demand for some CFA services (Table 7-1).

The primary service area is distinctly different from the remainder of D.C. Virtually all of the residents are black. There is a disproportionate number of young people in the area. Educational attainments of adults (over 25 years old) are dramatically lower than for the city as a whole. Not surprisingly, related findings reflected low housing values, limited home ownership, and a very large number of families living at or below the poverty level (Table 7-2).

Organizational Environment

The Greater Southeast Community Hospital Foundation, CFA's parent corporation, was established in 1955. Its purpose was to meet the need for an acute care hospital in this area. The hospital opened its doors in 1966. During this ten-year interval, however, changes elsewhere in the city precipitated the migration of many poor residents into the Anacostia area. This influx led to the emigration of many middle class, predominantly white, families. The board and managers of the hospital and its foundation changed also.

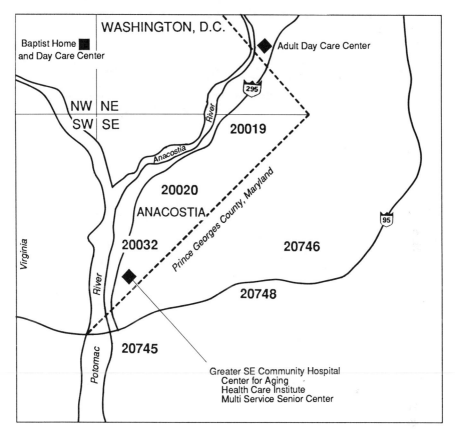

Exhibit 7-1 Washington, D.C. and surrounding area served by CFA.

The new leaders saw a need for a much broader mission if it was truly to meet the needs of the community. This vision was translated into three principal goals:

1. to provide an integrated system of comprehensive health services;

2. to support the economic redevelopment of the community;

3. to undertake sufficient profit generating activities to provide funds required for fulfillment of the Foundation's first two purposes.

Table 7-1 Percent of Greater Southeast Center for Aging clients residing in principal service areas.

Service	Areas and Zip Codes	
	Anacostia (20019,20020,20032)	PG County (20745,20746,20748)
Inpatient LTC	47 percent	1 percent
Day care	60 percent	8 percent
Community services[*]	63 percent	27 percent
Transportation	61 percent	24 percent
Assessment/case management**	95 percent	--

[*]Includes recreation, nutrition, and socialization
**Funded by D.C. Office on Aging

Source: Center for the Aging Patient Origin 1985, prepared by Planning Department, Greater Southeast Management Company.

These decisions led to the evolution of a health services system including the foundation, its management company, and six major subsidiaries (Exhibit 7-2). The Greater Southeast Management Company performed corporate functions for the entire system. The other major units and their roles follow.

Greater Southeast Community Hospital is a 450 bed acute-care facility with one of the busiest emergency departments in the city. The hospital had a number of special care units including intensive care, neonatal intensive care, psychiatric care, and home health care services.

Office Services Corporation, founded in 1978, is the business development subsidiary of the foundation. Its mission is to help meet the service and economic needs of the foundation and the community through the development of profit-making enterprises. Its operations include a medical office building, durable medical equipment rental and sales, pharmacies, and television rentals for hospital inpatients.

Fort Washington Ambulatory Care Center began operation in 1983 as an outpatient surgical facility offering a wide variety of services. In addition to the on-site surgical services, it also provides home health care as an outreach to the community.

Prefercare was organized in 1984 as the first preferred provider organization (PPO) in the Washington metropolitan area. It was created as a joint venture between private physicians and the Greater Southeast Community Hospital.

Parkwood Hospital, acquired in 1986, is a 33 bed facility with two operating rooms, radiology, laboratory and pharmacy services. It also operates an emergency room and a walk-in care center. The acute care provided at Parkwood focuses on geriatric care and in/out surgery.

The Greater Southeast Center for the Aging, (CFA), the other subsidiary, was a natural outgrowth of the foundation's decision to expand its mission. It was clear that the inadequacy of health care for elderly residents was a critical concern within the community. The foundation's leaders, however, saw that this was only part of the problem. By taking a systems perspective, they identified the need for a comprehensive center that could provide a full continuum of services needed by senior citizens.

The wisdom of this decision was recognized by a planning grant from the federal Administration on Aging which was attempting to foster development of integrated service systems. Further confirmation was provided by information gathered from the community as part of the initial planning process. These data showed that citizens felt that the need for a broad range of outpatient services was at least as great as the need for inpatient long term-care.

Characteristics	Zip Areas*			Total	CFA Service Area**	District of Columbia**
	20019	20020	20032			
Age						
Under 18 years	21,744	15,706	14,980	52,430	30%	24%
18 to 65	41,465	46,735	24,176	112,376	64%	64%
Over 65	5,467	4,805	1,637	11,909	7%	12%
Total	68,676	67,246	40,793	176,715		
Race						
Black	67,956	62,047	39,436	169,439	96%	70%
Other	344	494	346	1,184	1%	3%
White	376	4,705	1,011	6,092	3%	27%
School Completed						
0-11 years	17,394	14,817	7,931	40,142	43%	33%
12 years	12,810	12,737	7,832	33,379	36%	25%
13-15 years	4,190	5,281	2,774	12,245	13%	14%
16 or more years	2,490	3,767	1,291	7,548	8%	28%

The Need for a Client Data Base / 125

Characteristics	Zip Areas*				CFA Service Area**	District of Columbia**
	20019	20020	20032	Total		
Families						
In poverty	25%	25%	27%		25%	16%
Housing						
Owner occupied	32%	30%	17%		28%	35%
Housing values						
$50,000-99,999	42%	57%	26%		39%	18%
$100,000-149,999	49%	43%	71%		56%	49%
$150,000-199,999	7%	0%	0%		4%	15%
over $200,000	0%	0%	0%		0%	9%
Income						
Median family	$14276	$15,251	$15,812	n/a		$19,099
Per capita	$5667	$6,006	$5,326	n/a		$12,210

*Source: Service Area analyses prepared by planning Department of Greater Southeast Management Co.
**Source: *Indices*, July 1986; prepared by D.C. Office of Policy and Program Evaluation.

Exhibit 7-2 Greater Southeast Community Hospital Foundation Organizational Chart.

The CFA Philosophy

Every organization has a driving force, a set of values that dominates in all major decisions and, hopefully, permeates day-by-day operations. The driving force of the Foundation clearly was community service. In CFA there was also an exceptionally strong commitment to provision of quality care which emphasized the dignity of each individual. Two examples illustrate the effects of this conviction. Nurse staffing in inpatient facilities was maintained at a level well above that required by government regulations despite reimbursement based on the prescribed minimum level of staffing. Housekeeping carried out an unusually aggressive, continuous cleaning program so none of the typical unpleasant environmental conditions (e.g., odors) were ever found in CFA facilities.

The Evolution of the CFA

Although this driving force evolved over time, it was fostered by the original philosophy of complete community service. This philosophy was the basis for a four phase development plan.

Phase One focused on the case assessment/case management function and the senior activities center. It was also intended to include transportation, nutrition, pharmacy, home care, and home support services. Phase Two was the addition of medical adult day care and affiliations with a university. An inpatient nursing facility, a mental health program, and a gerontological research program were all part of Phase Three. Phase Four included the completion of 50 to 60 housing units for the elderly who would also be users of other center services as appropriate.

As is often the case, implementation did not follow the plan exactly. The first component of CFA was a senior activities program. This was followed closely by a project to construct an inpatient facility. The project was started promptly because the availability of long-term care beds could lead to more efficient use of acute care beds in the hospital and the facility construction process would last for at least one year. In fact, several problems delayed the facility's occupancy for more than two years.

Meanwhile, there was considerable progress being made on the other phases. Trained social workers were added to the Senior Center's staff. Thus, it was possible to inaugurate the case assessment/case management function. Also, transportation services and nutrition programs began. Next, a medical day care program was

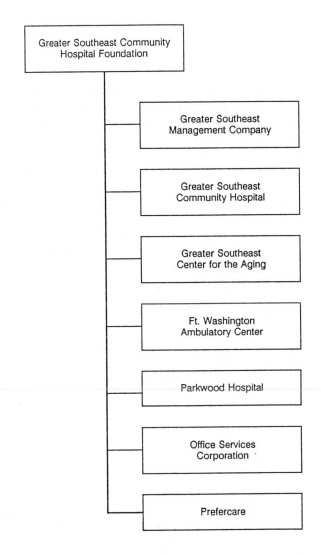

Exhibit 7-2 Greater Southeast Community Hospital Foundation Organizational Chart.

established. At this point, the senior center was appropriately renamed as the Multi-Service Senior Center (MSSC). Later, MSSC services were again expanded to include outreach and counseling and a special program to assist recently discharged mental patients. The latter, designated as the Saturday Socialization Program, was established in collaboration with Saint Elizabeth's Hospital, a mental health facility, to strengthen its deinstitutionalization program.

When the inpatient facility was dedicated, it was named The Health Care Institute (HCI). The early years following the opening of HCI brought the realization that financial viability would not be achieved easily. This was attributed to two facts. First, HCI rapidly reached 100 percent occupancy, but virtually all of the residents were Medicaid beneficiaries rather than private pay patients. Second, Medicaid would not fully reimburse HCI for the level of nursing care consistent with CFA's philosophy.

Initial efforts to change the payor mix were relatively unsuccessful. Consequently, CFA rethought its business strategy. It accepted the fact that its commitment to serve the community inevitably caused it to be a "Medicaid facility." Concurrently, it became more entrepreneurial and sought opportunities to engage in revenue generating activities.

This strategy was successful in that CFA won contracts to manage two major programs. The first contract made CFA responsible for the management of the Stoddard Baptist Home, a 164 bed intermediate care nursing facility located in northwest D.C. (ZIP code area 20011 on Exhibit 7-1). The second contract obligated CFA to establish and operate an adult day care program for senior citizens of Prince Georges County. This activity is housed in the Cora B. Woods Senior Center, Brentwood, Maryland (ZIP code area 20722 on Exhibit 7-1). Despite these successes, which eventually contributed to a sound financial base for operations, CFA sources of revenues remained unbalanced. Inpatient services generated 91 percent of all revenues and Medicaid provided 85 percent of all payments.

Throughout its history, CFA has been aggressive and successful in seeking grants to support its innovative programs. Much of this activity was carried out by its unique organizational component, the Office of Research, Education and Training (RET). The first major grant was awarded to CFA by The Robert Wood Johnson Foundation to support the development of a teaching nursing home as an analog to a teaching hospital. The goal was to establish a partnership between a university and a nursing home that would lead to enhanced quality of care and improved geriatric education, particularly for medical and nursing students. The second grant of national significance supported establishment of a Service Credit Volunteer System (SCVS). The system's goal was to offer older people an opportunity to provide as well as to receive services.

Participants provide services to others and, in exchange, receive credits which they could use to purchase services for themselves. For example, a person with an automobile might provide transportation to earn credits that could be used to get assistance with home repairs. An additional CFA component, a 69-unit housing project, was in the construction phase. This was possible because CFA helped to secure a HUD 202 grant, the first awarded for the Anacostia area. The size and scope of the CFA programs are detailed by the data in Table 7-3.

The CFA Board

Although CFA was a subsidiary of the foundation, it was governed by its own board of directors. The CFA board was composed of persons representing both political jurisdictions (D.C. and Prince Georges County) served by its programs. These members included service providers and professionals in aging, business persons, and consumers. The members provided the organization with a wide range of expertise.

Each of the directors served on at least one of the board committees. This arrangement had been designed to maximize the effectiveness of each member's strengths in providing direction to the center. In addition to its regular meetings, the board held at least one annual retreat to evaluate the year's performance, to identify new goals, and to develop a plan of action.

The CFA Management Structure

Initially, CFA was a small organization managed through very informal arrangements. As it grew, the leaders recognized the need for more structured interaction to ensure proper allocations of authority and responsibility. A matrix management structure was adopted. The organization's history of informality and shared responsibility and the belief that such a structure would be compatible with and supportive of the CFA patient care philosophy were the reasons behind the choice of this structure.

Gradually, however, CFA moved toward a more traditional, hierarchical management structure. This change took place as a result of several factors. High staff turnover made it difficult to maintain the high level of individual expertise required for acceptance of broad responsibility. This turnover also included the key

Table 7-3 Scope of Services provided by CFA programs.

The following are quantitative data for CFA programs.

Health Care Institute (HCI) annual data
- Beds: 180 ICF
- Patient days: 64,683
- Occupancy rate: 98.7 percent
- Meals served: 230,048
- Therapy visits: 3,259
- Scheduled activities: 1,669
- Employees: 245 FTEs
- Average length of stay: 2 years
- Discharge rate: 10 percent discharged to community
- Reimbursement: 95 percent Medicaid, 3 percent Private, 2 percent Medicare

Stoddard Baptist Nursing Home (current data)
- Beds: 164 ICF
- Occupancy rate: 90 percent after 6 months under CFA management
- Employees: 132 FTEs (The apparent discrepancy in staffing levels between Stoddard and HCI was attributable to the fact that Stoddard performed many functions with contract labor: e.g., dietary and housekeeping)

Brentwood Medical Adult Day Care Center (current data)
- Average census: 17 people (30 enrollees)
- Capacity: census of 27 (50 enrollees)
- Average stay: 6-8 hours/day, 5 days/week
- Reimbursement: Medicaid and private pay

Multi-Service Senior Center - (MSSC) annual data*
- Medical day care: 4,889 participant days (50 enrollees)
- Community program: 12,330 participant days (250 enrollees)
- Congregate meals: 20,250 Served (300 enrollees)
- Transportation program: 12,123 People (100 enrollees)
- Community outreach and counseling program: 1,316 Units (75 enrollees)
- Assessment/case management: 4,116 units (135 enrollees)
- Saturday socialization program: 878 Participant Days (20 enrollees)
- Senior companion program: 4,019 visits (not considered enrollees)
- Employees: 27 FTE's

* Many persons were enrolled in several programs; e.g., meals, community program and transportation.

Service Credit Volunteer System SCVS current data
- Participants: 125 people

proponents of the matrix model and these people were replaced by individuals who saw greater advantages in more traditional management approaches.   Diversification and growth of CFA programs made it increasingly difficult to maintain the necessary levels of coordination and accountability.

Eventually, the CFA management structure was comprised of two major operating elements and two principal staff offices, all of which reported directly to the president. (The president of CFA was also a vice-presidents in the Greater Southeast Management Company). The CFA vice-president for inpatient services was responsible for the two nursing homes, HCI and Stoddard. The responsibilities of the other vice-presidents included all outpatient services (MSSC and the Brentwood ADHC program). The staff offices were Finance and Program and Human Development. The latter office was responsible for overseeing the activities of Research, Education and Training, Service Credit Volunteer Service, and the CFA personnel office (Exhibit 7-3).

Despite the hierarchical nature of the formal organization, CFA retained many of the features of its earlier matrix structure. This can be illustrated with two examples. The CFA president held regular monthly meetings in which vice-presidents, staff directors, and program managers participated on an equal footing. Communications flowed directly and easily across organizational boundaries for tasks requiring collaborative effort.

This situation was reinforced by the management style of CFA's leaders. The president and vice-presidents were adept practitioners of what Peters and Waterman (1982) call "management by wandering around."

The Lack of Services Integration

A year ago the president of the foundation became concerned about the integration of services provided by components of the corporation, particularly with regard to the needs of the elderly. The acute care hospital had made some efforts to ensure that this was happening. It had established a multi-disciplinary geriatric team to coordinate its services. But how should this interface with the services offered by CFA? A consultant's study commissioned by the foundation concluded there was a "lack of inter-affiliate referrals" attributable to a lack of structure. This finding led to a recommendation for appointment of a program director and a geriatric care and quality assurance committee at the corporate level. The new director and the committee would be responsible for guiding, coordinating, and monitoring the activities of two independent assessment and case management offices—one in the hospital and one in CFA.

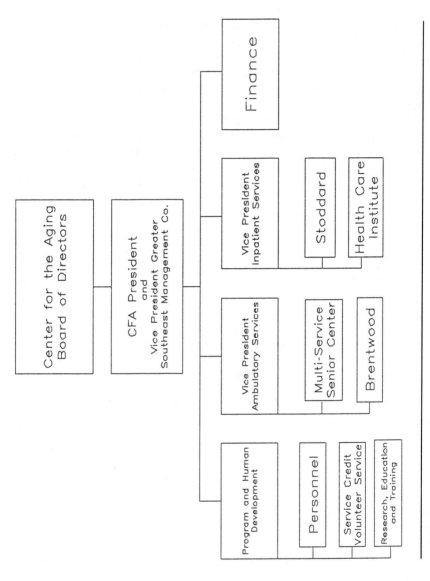

Exhibit 7-3 Center for the Aging Organizational Chart.

A staff review of the consultant's report indicated that it was based largely upon a few unrepresentative interviews and so was not an accurate portrayal of the existing situation. The staff also felt strongly that the proposed organizational change would lead to an expensive, but ineffective, addition to the foundation's management structure.

In an effort to develop positive recommendations, a geriatric services task force made up of representatives of the hospital and CFA staffs conducted a survey of all system components that served the elderly. An additional focus of the survey was data being collected by each component. Exhibits 7-4 through 7-12 contain representations of the forms used by various components of CFA. These forms were collected because a fundamental premise of the task force was that a unified automated data system would serve several important purposes. These were:

1. Create a complete inventory of persons using services of the system,

2. Identify persons receiving services from more than one component,

3. Facilitate and track movement of clients among the components of the system,

4. Reduce duplicate data collection and storage, and

5. Provide information system support to managers of all service components.

A number of programs had no automated information and relied entirely upon manual data collection, storage, and manipulation.

Information Systems Configuration

CFA had a variety of data processing arrangements and only one trained systems analyst. The equipment was distributed as follows among CFA components.

CFA Corporate Offices (located in ZIP code 20748 on Exhibit 7-1)
Two dedicated terminals for a brand X proprietary financial
management system
Two IBM personal computers (1 PC; 1 XT)

CENTER FOR THE AGING
Washington, D.C.

Application for Admission

The Health Care Institute has agreed to comply with the provisions of the Civil Rights Act of 1964 and all requirements imposed pursuant thereto, to the end that no person shall, on the grounds of race, color, or national origin, be excluded from participation in, be denied benefits of, or otherwise be subject to discrimination in the provision of any care or service.

Directions: Part A is to be completed by the applicant or by a relative or friend.
Part B is to be completed by a social worker, nurse, or physician involved with the applicant's care.

Part A

Name _____

Address _____
Number   Street

_____
City   State   Zip code

Current location _____
If different
_____
_____

Telephone number _____

Responsible party: _____
Name

Address _____

_____

Telephone number _____

Date of application _____

Date of birth _____

Sex _____ Age _____

Marital status _____

Ethnic group _____
(For statistical purposes only)
Religion _____

Birthplace _____

Social security no. _____

Relationship

List other relatives and friends in the area:

Name	Relationship	Address	Telephone

Source of payment: Private pay   Yes_____   No_____

Medicare no. _____ Medicaid No. _____

Other insurance: _____

Income source: _____

_____
_____

Exhibit 7-4 Application for admission to HCI. Source: Center for the Aging, Washington, D.C.

Services/care: Is the applicant currently receiving:

    Nursing services? No ____ Yes, from _____

    Physician services? No ____ Yes, from _____

    Personal care services? No ____ Yes, from _____

Please describe how family and friends are involved at the present time.

_____

_____

_____

Why are you applying to the Health Care Institute? _____

_____

_____

How long do you expect to reside at the HCI? 2 weeks or less_____ 2-4 weeks___ 1-3 months___ 3-6 months___

6 months or more_____

Have you visited the HCI? Yes____ No___ If not, would you like to?

When would be the best time for you? _____

I hearby apply for admission to the Health Care Institute and certify that all the information furnished is factual, accurate, and without omission or misrepresentation.

_____   _____

          Date   Signature

If not signed by the applicant, what is your relationship?_____
Is the applicant aware that this application is being made?
        Yes_____No, because _____

Part B: To be completed be a social worker, nurse, or physician who is currently involved in the applicant's care

Applicant's name _____ Date _____

Informant's name _____ Phone _____
                                           (daytime please)

Title _____

Address _____

Certified level of care _____

1. Eating
    ____Independent
    ____With assistance
    ____Spoon feeding
    ____Tube feeding

2. Ambulation
    ____Independent
    ____With assistance
    ____With device_____ (specify)
    ____Does not ambulate

3. Transfer
    ____Independent
    ____With assistance
    ____Dependent

4. Continence
    Bowel: Y__N__Some_____
    Bladder: Y__N__Some_____
    Catheter:_____
               (specify)

Exhibit 7-4, continued.

5. Skin integrity (decubitus)
   Number_____
   Size_____
   Location_____

6. Mental
   ___Oriented
   ___Somewhat disoriented
   ___Highly disoriented
   ___Comatose

7. Supervision needed
   ___None
   ___Occasionally
   ___Frequently
   ___Constantly

8. Behavior
   ___Cooperative
   ___Combative
   ___Wanders
   _____

9. Medically stable
   ___Yes
   ___No,_____
   _____

10. Other treatments
    ___OT/PT Rx___x/week
    ___O^2 _____suctioning
    _____

11. Diagnosis list
    _____
    _____
    _____

12. Recent surgery and date:_____

13. Hospitalizations in the past 2 years. Include facility, reason, and length of stay._____
    _____
    _____
    _____

14. Current medications (list)_____
    _____
    _____

15. Rehabilitation potential: Yes___ No___explain either._____
    _____

16. Indicate date and results of these tests:

    TB Skin Test_____ _____ Chest x-ray _____ _____
           (date)   (result)   (date)   (result)

    VDRL _____ _____
         (date)   (result)

17. Has the applicant been referred to the Central Referral Bureau?
    Yes, on _____ No_____

18. Name and address of physician if additional information is needed.
    _____
    _____

19. Additional comments on (family or other social supports, other relevant information).
    _____
    _____
    _____

Date_____ Signature_____

Exhibit 7-4, continued.

CENTER FOR AGING
Washington, D.C.

THE HEALTH CARE INSTITUTE
FINANCIAL ADMISSION/DISCHARGE FORM

Code	Client ID	Patient no.	Time of admission	AM PM

Top for business office use only		Attach copy of MC/MA card		

Admit date	Patient type	Level of Care S or I	Room number	

Patient's last name	First name	Middle initial	Birth date	Sex

Patient address (for billing info.)

Birth place (City, State)	Occupation	Marital status	Religion	Age

Father's name		Mother's name		Relationship of guarantor

Guarantor's name	Guarantor's home address

Guarantor's home phone	Guarantor's bus. phone

Notify in emergency- first preference	Home phone	Bus. phone

Second preference	Home phone	Bus. phone

Soc. sec. no.	Medicare Policy or Med. Assist no.	Bill override

Eligible for Medicare Part B Y or N	Part B coins. acct. type	Medicare days left	Coinsurance rate

Third party type code		Welfare no.	Medicaid no.

Private portion	Contract rate	Code	Auto misc./charge codes

Sponsoring organization or state agency

Physician name	Lic. no.	Address	Phone

Admitting diagnosis-1	Admitting diagnosis -2

Name and address of qualifying hospital stays

Date last hosp. admit	Date last hosp. disch.	Medicare status	Prolonged care

Notes:

Do Not Write Below This Line

Discharge Information

Discharge date Expired Y or N	Discharge number	Discharge code

Discharge diagnosis-1	Discharge diagnosis-2

Discharged by	Time of discharge

Patient's forwarding address

Exhibit 7-5 HCI financial admission/discharge form.

Assessment Visit Report

CENTER FOR THE AGING
Washington, D.C.

Name_____
DOB_____
Current placement_____
( ) Home ( ) CRF ( ) Hosp. ( ) Nursing home monthly income ( ) $400 ( ) $400 +
Admission date_____

Total LOC score_____
Date/initial assessment_____
Level of care_____

Note: Check appropriate category

Item	1	2	3	
Feeding	Independent	Assistance	Spoon feeding/NG/G tube	
Personal Care (bathing/dressing)	Independent/needs direction	Needs assistance	Totally dependent	Physician:
Mobility	Independent/device	Assist with wheeling walking	Bedfast/chairfast transfer/wheeling	VDRL: Chest x-ray:
Psychosocial management	Oriented/occasionally disoriented; cooperative; occasional to no supervision	Partially dis-oriented: con-fused; frequent supervision	Totally disoriented wanders/combative/screams; constant supervision	Family support:
Continency	Continent of U&F; infrequent incontinence	Frequent incon-tinence bowel/bladder	Total incontinence bowel/bladder colostomy/catheter	

Skin Integrity	Intact	Superficial lesions	Deep lesions
Monitoring Requirement	Routine	Expected intermittent	Constant
Diagnosis	–	–	New DX
Surgery	–	–	Recent
Medications	0-2	3-5 or- psychotrophic drugs	6+ or insulin
Rehab. Potential	–	Yes/ROM	–

( ) Foley   ( ) Colostomy   ( ) Rehab. potential ( ) Yes ( ) No
( ) Decubiti: #_____   Size_____   Location_____

Special Services (check all which apply)
( ) Dialysis ( ) Trach   ( ) Respirator   ( ) Communicable disease
( ) IV ( ) O2 ( ) Severe behavior disturbance ( ) Terminal illness
( ) Acute illness ( ) Frequent suctioning Age: _____ <60   _____ 60 +

Diagnosis (list; include h/o Etoh):   Medications (lists);

Exhibit 7-6 Assessment visit report. Source: Center for the Aging, Washington, D.C.

CENTER FOR THE AGING
Washington, D.C.

Social Information and Background Data

1.   Name_____ Admission date_____

2.   Address prior to nursing home admission_____

2a.   Home address, if different_____

3.   Other places of residence_____

4a.   Birthdate and place of birth_____

4b.   Father's name_____4c. Mother's name_____

5.   Where did resident live <u>most</u> of adult life?_____

6.   Education_____

7.   Occupation_____7a. Main jobs_____

8.   Marriage date_____
      a. Spouse's name, age, address_____

      b. Divorced, widowed - If yes, the date_____
      c. Describe the important characteristic of the marriage(s)_____

      d. Is the resident especially sensitive about any aspects of the marriage(s). How has this been handled?_____

9a.   Names of resident's living brothers and sisters and present contacts and relationship with them.
      (1)_____

      (2)_____

9b.   Total number of siblings_____

10.   Children's names and addresses and present contacts and relationship with resident.
      (1)_____

      (2)_____

11.   Other significant people, such as close friends, other relatives, etc., and their present contacts and relationship with residents.
      _____

      Whom does the resident trust most? The least?_____

1.   What is the resident's usual temperament or disposition?_____

2.   Is this behavior different from the past? If so, describe using examples._____

3.   How has he/she reacted to losses, such as death of a loved one, moving, or separations from family, especially recent losses?_____

4.   Describe how any problems have been managed. With what results?_____

5.   What problems can we expect? Suggestions for handling?_____

Exhibit 7-7 Social information and background data form. Source: Center for the Aging, Washington, D.C.

1. What has he been told about his condition and outlook for the future? His reaction?_____

2. What has the resident been told about coming into the home? His reaction?

3. Describe in your own words why resident is coming into the home. Include details that you consider significant.____

4. Who or what was most influential in making the final decision and how did this come about?_____

5. In the event the resident improves sufficently to be discharged, is there a tentative plan? What family members are, will be involved in the planning?_____

6. Medical evaluation_____

7. Physical deformities or limitations_____

---

1. Foreign places lived in _____Where traveled_____
2. Foreign languages_____Read?_____Speak?_____
3. Spectator activities
   ( ) Sports   ( ) Reading   Note:_____
   ( ) Movies, plays   ( ) Radio   _____
   ( ) TV   ( ) Other   _____

4. Participating activites
   ( ) Sports   ( ) Walking   Note:_____
   ( ) Cards   _alone   _____
   ( ) Games   _with/assist.   _____
   ( ) Visit w/friends _non-ambulatory
   ( ) Letterwriting

5. Hobbies and creative arts
   ( ) Sew or handwork ( ) Music   Note:_____
   ( ) Crafts   ( ) Dance   _____
   ( ) Gardening   ( ) Pets   _____

6. Church
   Denomination_____Name of church_____
   Minister_____
   Would you like local minister to be notified?_____
   No church interest or affilation_____

7. Lodges, clubs, veterans organizations, politics, other community activities. Name and describe activity_____

8. Any activities which patient no longer does, which might be renewed with encouragement_____

   Anything always wanted to try but never got around to?_____

9. Comments:

Exhibit 7-7, continued.

CENTER FOR THE AGING
Washington, DC

Nursing Data Base

Name of informant:_____

I. Identifying data:
    a. Admission date_____ b. Religious affiliation_____
    c. Previous occupation_____
    d. Family/support system_____
        _____
    e. Medical DX_____
    f. Allergies (food, medicine, environmental)_____
    g. General appearance/health status/self image: hgt._____ wgt._____
        _____
        _____

II. Universal self-care requisites:

    a. Air (SOB, TBc, Smoking, COPD)_____
    b. Food (appetite, preferences, allergies, difficulty swallowing/digestion, dentures_____
    c. Water (hydration status/skin turgor, IVs)_____
    d. Elimination (constipation, hemorrhoids, impaction, diarrhea, flatulance, continence, use of toilet/appliances,
        hygiene/ grooming)_____
    e. Activity (mobility, independence/limitation, prosthesis, assistive device, e.g., cane/wc/walker, tolerance level,
        activities, interests)_____
    f. Rest (sleep/rest pattern, aids)_____
        _____
    g. Solitude (need for) _____
        _____
    h. Social interaction (relationships, communication problems)_____
        _____
    i. Protection from hazards (hx falls, alcohol/drug abuse, need for side rails,_____
    j. Normalcy (what is healthy about self? Special strengths and interests)_____
    k. Managing disorders (meds, treatments) _____
        _____

III. Summarize resident concerns:_____
     _____

IV. Summarize family interests and concerns regarding resident:
    _____
    _____
    _____
    _____

Date_____ Nurse signature_____

Exhibit 7-8 Nursing data base form. Source: Center for the Aging, Washington, D.C.

Health Care Institute
Transfer Form

Transferred from: Transferred to:
   The Health Care Institute _____
   Washington, D.C. _____
                          _____

Patient name:_____

Private ECF _____Medicare_n____ Medicaid_____VA_____

Medicare no._____   Social security no._____

Medicaid no._____   VA no._____

Date of birth:_____   Sex:_____ Marital status:_____

Responsible party:_____   Relationship:_____

Address:_____   Phone:_____
_____
_____

Immediate problem:_____

Medical problems:_____   Drugs/diet/nursing_____
_____   _____
_____   _____

Allergies: Y__N__specify:_____

Primary nurse:_____   MD (signature)_____
Phone_____   Phone_____

Findings/recommendations: Fill out and return to HCI.

Expected length of stay:_____ Signature/date_____

Exhibit 7-9 HCI transfer form.

Health Care Institute
Medical Discharge Summary

1. Resident name_____ Adm. no._____ DOB_____

2. Room no._____ Age_____

3. Diagnoses (1)_____ (2)_____
   (3)_____

4. Functional prognosis: ___Improving ___Stable ___Declining

5. Summary, course of treatment while in HCI_____
   _____
   _____

6. Resident discharged: Alive _____ Dead_____
   If discharged dead: Time of death____ Date of death_____
   Name of funeral home:_____

7. Proposed treatment plan_____
   _____
   _____
   _____

8. Physician orders_____
   _____
   _____

9. Sponsor of next of kin to whom resident discharged:
   Name and relationship_____
   Address_____
   Phone_____

10. Resident discharged by: ____ Ambulance ____ Wheelchair
    (choose two)   ____ Priv. trans. ____ Ambulatory
                             ____ Stretcher   ____ Assistance

11. Patient condition at discharge_____
    _____

12. Primary physician_____

13. Attending physician_____
    Address_____
    Phone_____

Summary completed by: (signature) _____M.D.

Date _____

Exhibit 7-10 HCI medical discharge summary form.

CENTER FOR THE AGING
Washington, D.C.

Brentwood Medical Adult Daycare
Admission Assessment

Date_____
D.O.B._____

Name: _____   Social security:_____

Address: _____   Marital status:_____

_____

Phone: _____   Alternate phone:_____

Physician: _____   Phone:_____

Address: _____

_____

Date of last checkup:_____Other insurance:_____

I. Living arrangements: House_____(or) Apt._____Stairs_____

Number of people:_____ (List with relationship)
1. _____
2. _____

Name, day phone, and address of other family members or friends:
1. _____
2. _____

II. Social history

Brief history of location:_____

Education:_____
Other agencies involved:_____
Date and circustances of retirement:_____
Patient's or family's goals:_____
Activities, interests:_____

III. Medical history

Diagnoses:_____

Medications:_____

Diet:_____

Physical limitations:_____

Alergies:_____
Hospitalizations:_____
Accidents or injuries:_____

Exhibit 7-11 Admission assessment form (Brentwood Medical Adult Daycare). Source: Center for the Aging, Washington, D.C.

CENTER FOR AGING
Washington, D.C.

Multi–Service Senior Center/Day Care Program
Admission Assessment

Date_____
D.O.B._____

Name:_____
Address: _____   Social security_____
_____   Marital status_____
Phone: _____   Alternate phone:_____
Physician:_____   Phone:_____
Address:_____
Date of last checkup:_____Other insurance:_____

I. Living arrangements: House_____(or) Apt._____Stairs_____

Number of people:_____ (List with relationship)
1. _____
2. _____
Name, day phone and address of other family members or friends:
1. _____
_____
2. _____
_____

II. Social history

Brief history of location:_____
_____
Education: _____
Occupations:_____
Other agencies involved:_____
Date and circumstances of retirement:_____
Patient's or family's goals:_____
Activites, interests:_____

III. Medical history

Diagnoses:_____
_____
Medications:_____
Diet:_____
_____
Physical limitations:_____
_____
Allergies:_____
Hospitalizations:_____
Accidents or injuries:_____

IV. Psychosocial

Concerns, preoccupations_____
Depressions, fears, anger_____
_____
Recent losses – last 2 years_____
_____
Psychiatric treatment_____
_____

V. Mental status

A. Time, date, year, month, season
B. Place
C. Person and family
D. Remote memory
E. Recent memory

Exhibit 7-12 Admission assessment form (Multi-Service Senior Center/Day Care Program). Source: Center for the Aging, Washington, D.C.

Stoddard Nursing Home
Two dedicated terminals for a brand Y proprietary financial
management system
One IBM personal computer (AT)

HCI
Two IBM personal computers (XT)
One Radio Shack personal computer (for word processing)

SCVS (located in the HCI building)
One IBM personal computer dedicated to operation of that
program's record keeping using a preprogrammed data base
management system

MSSC
No computers

Brentwood
No computers

Spreadsheet, data base management, and word processing
software packages were available for all IBM personal computers.
Information was transmitted among CFA sites by a courier who
made two deliveries each working day. There was also a modem
linkage between the CFA corporate office and the finance office at
Stoddard Nursing Home. When necessary, information could be
hand carried among all sites. Round trip time between corporate
office, MSSC, and HCI was 20 minutes or less. Round trips from
any of these sites to Stoddard or Brentwood required approximately
50 minutes.

The hospital had a large mainframe computer with a staff of
trained analysts, programmers, and operators. The equipment and
staff supported many complex operations including hospital financial
management and corporate personnel management. CFA was in
the process of converting its personnel management system from a
free-standing, contractor-operated system to the corporate system.
The long-range data processing plans included development of a
client data system to serve all organizations within the foundation.
The plan, however, indicated that such a system would not be
implemented for at least three years. Many people thought this was
a very optimistic estimate.

The CFA Decision—An Interim System

Top management of CFA felt that this schedule was unacceptable. They had an immediate need for client information to support day-to-day operations, strategic planning, and research. On the other hand, they could not afford to commit their scarce resources to a costly interim system which would be discarded when the corporate system came on-line.

As a consequence of this dilemma, a decision was made to develop and implement an interim system based on certain criteria which would minimize anticipated negative effects. The system should be:

1. Based on personal computer technology since CFA already had six PC's and since any additions to existing hardware capacity would be inexpensive.

2. Very "user friendly" so the staff could use it without extensive training.

3. Flexible and easy for the staff to modify in order to incorporate lessons learned as they became experienced users.

4. Compatible with other systems. It should allow easy exchange of information with other computer programs such as spreadsheets and the proposed corporate client data system.

5. Responsive to management needs. It should be able to provide prompt answers to specific questions. In other words, the system's output should be rapid responses to individual management queries rather than general purpose reports produced on a periodic cycle.

Management needed additional information to develop this interim system. The first step was to define the data base (Part A):

1. What data elements should be required for all persons participating in any of CFA's programs?

2. What additional program-specific data elements should be required for persons enrolled in each CFA program?

3. How should each data element be recorded to ensure consistency among CFA components and between CFA and external agencies? For example, activities of daily living (ADL) scales should be uniform within CFA. They should also be compatible with the requirements of a reimbursement system based on resource utilization groups (RUGs) which was being developed by one of the Medicaid offices.

The next step involved hardware/software selection (Part B):

1. What criteria should be used in selecting the hardware and software configuration for the CFA client data base system?

2. What alternative configurations are feasible? (These configurations should be developed using descriptions of currently available hardware and software.)

3. What is the best configuration for CFA?

Another consideration was the ongoing operation of the system (Part C):

1. What criteria should be used to evaluate the operation of an information system of this nature?

2. What specific functions must be performed to satisfy these criteria?

3. Where should responsibilities for these functions be placed within the organization?

4. What staffing is required to carry out these functions?

Finally, it was necessary to plan for implementation (Part D):

1. What activities are required to implement the CFA client data base system?

2. What resources are required to carry out these activities?

3. What should be the schedule for implementing the system?

4. How should CFA management ensure that the implementation is accomplished on schedule?

Case 8

Capturing Lost Charges: Tranquility Health Care Center*

Richard Brown

Richard Brown, M.H.A., is Assistant Professor/Coordinator, Division of Health Care Management, Florida A&M University.

The following situations exemplify the state of affairs at Tranquility Health Care Center (THCC) during this past summer. They all involve the occurrence of unwanted expenses and raise the issue of organizational efficiency and effectiveness. To improve the situations, good managerial problem solving and decision making are required.

Situation 1

At 11:35 A.M. Shirley Nelson, a dietary aide, just completed loading the food cart and hurriedly pushed it through the dining room door and down a hall. As Shirley rushed the cart past the activity room, she took a left turn at the end of the corridor to arrive at the sitting area in front of the nurses' station, announcing, "Lunch is here." Two of six nursing assistants responded immediately. They opened doors, looking up and down the cart as they check the names of residents. The other four aides arrived about two minutes later.

---

* Fictitious names of both the organization and individuals are used to ensure anonymity.

151

The first nursing assistant pulled one of the food trays from the cart in a routine manner and hurried over to a shiny stainless steel utility cart. Removing the cellophane covering from the plastic cup, she emptied the contents into the trash bag on the cart. She then uncovered the dessert and the main dish, and with a fork she raked the contents into the trash bag. When she had thrown away the entire meal she stacked the dishes neatly on the second shelf of the utility cart. She then rushed back to the food cart to remove a second tray. Immediately she repeated the process of throwing away another entire meal. Yet again she returned to the food cart, took out a third tray, and repeated the strange action.

Situation 2

It was Dorothy Jackson's second day on the job as a nursing assistant. She asked Rita Picco, who had been employed for one week, "What are those little white stickers that I'm seeing all over the place?"

"I think those are stickers that came off the supplies used for the residents," replied Rita.

"Oh. Okay. I was wondering about them because I have seen them sticking on the nursing station counter, the I.V. poles, on the fronts and backs of charts . . . they're everywhere!"

"I know what you mean. I've seen them sticking on the nurses' uniforms and on the utility carts. I even saw a bunch of them in the trash once. But don't worry about them now. We'll learn about them when we go through orientation. Right now our most important job is to take good care of the residents we're assigned."

Situation 3

It was 3:30 P.M. on a Thursday afternoon and Nicky Bolden, who is the ward clerk responsible for medical records and purchasing (and reports to the director of nursing services), was making a telephone call.

"Hello, this is Nicky Bolden at Tranquility Health Care Center. . . . Yes, it's me again. We would like to place an ad in your paper for nursing assistants. Do you have a copy of what we used a couple months ago? . . . OK, good. We would like to run the same copy for the next three weekends. Just bill us as usual. How much will the ad cost? . . . What? Why is that? What do you mean we have to send a check for $600.00 before you can run the ad? . . . You mean we have an outstanding balance from a couple months ago? . . . OK, I'll talk to the director of nursing and the administrator about it and get back with you."

Nicky hung up the phone, grumbling to herself, "Hmmmph! Isn't this something. Here we are, short of nurses' aides, the new nursing wing is supposed to open in two weeks, and we can't even place an ad because corporate headquarters hasn't paid the bill for two months now."

Overview

Tranquility Health Care Center is a 120-bed facility with 24-hour licensed skilled nursing care. Located in the southeastern part of the United States, in the Sun Belt, the complex sits in a quiet wooded area on a 5-acre tract surrounded by tall pines and palm trees. The average annual temperature of the area is 68 degrees. The community hospital is located less than half a mile down the winding road to the west of THCC. The area is served by two hospitals with over 900 beds providing acute care to permanent residents and to the student population. The center is located in a medium-sized city with a population of 125,000 and a county population of 180,000. Two universities, one junior college, and a vocational school are located in the city. The city enjoys a stable economy, with primary employers that include state government and educational institutions. The largest private employer is one of the hospitals.

There are five nursing homes located in the area, and two of them are located within two miles of THCC. The administrator is not particularly concerned about the competition. She believes that THCC is the flagship nursing home in the area. She does keep informed about a certain nursing home near THCC that opened a year ago. Already it has received poor publicity concerning quality of care issues.

The History of Tranquility Health Care Center

The center was opened in February 1980 by a local company that operated the center for approximately two years. From its start, the organization was plagued by a reputation for problems between administration and personnel. These problems were reflected in less than desirable care provided to residents. Care for the majority of residents was paid by Medicaid while only 5 percent of the clients paid with personal funds. Two administrators occupied the primary leadership position during this time.

In 1981, the facility was purchased by a national nursing home corporation with an established reputation for expertise in the long-term care industry. This company operated the facility for two years and during this time the nursing home grew from an average occupancy rate of 75 percent to 85 percent. The administrator who occupied the leadership position for these two years was considered strong and effective.

The facility's current owner is a relatively young company with more than 20 nursing homes across the United States. They assumed ownership of THCC four years ago. The corporation takes pride in living up to a philosophy that the quality of care and the success of the center is determined by the attitude and dedication of the employees. As reflected in its statement of philosophy toward residents and employees, the company is committed to helping residents achieve their fullest physical, emotional, and spiritual potential (Exhibit 8-1).

The current mix of residents based on payment source is as follows:

Private	42%
Medicaid	54%
V.A.	4%
Medicare	0%
	100%

Since the current owners purchased the center, the number of private pay residents has increased significantly. One of the goals of the corporation is to increase this proportion to 50 percent (other corporate goals are listed in Exhibit 8-2).

As a result of a continued 98 percent occupancy rate and the state health council's study of three years ago indicating need for additional long-term care beds in the area, THCC made plans to expand its capacity by 36 additional beds. The corporation felt that a new wing would allow the center to capture a greater share of the market. The certificate of need was applied for and granted two years ago. A groundbreaking ceremony took place a few months later. Several postponements have occurred in the opening date for the new wing. The original target date of late last year was changed to early this year, and then to the summer. Although the contractors completed their work by late summer, the construction has not yet

---

Policy Regarding Residents

1. Provide each resident professional care by a trained staff competent in recognizing and meeting each resident's needs.
2. Provide each resident the opportunity to live in an environment which will enhance their life style.
3. Acknowledge and endorse of the individual rights and respect every human deserves.
4. Develop techniques that will facilitate growth or change to a life style more compatible with the resident's needs and views.
5. Assist each resident to maintain the highest level of health, independence, and dignity.

Policy Regarding Employees

We view our employees as important members of our team. Therefore, we will strive to:

1. Treat employees fairly, with dignity as individuals, to avoid favoritism and to administer all policies, rules, and benefits consistently among employees.
2. Provide safe and orderly working conditions in all areas.
3. Train and guide employees and periodically keep them informed of their progress.
4. Invite constructive suggestions and criticism and guarantee the right to be heard without fear of reprisal.
5. Take all practical measures to solve problems affecting employees.
6. Give helpful consideration and guidance to employees.
7. Terminate employees only when there is good reason.
8. Keep employees informed of rules, policies, activities, and changes concerning their status.
9. Respect and support federal and local laws safeguarding the rights of employees.
10. Endeavor to offer good pay and competitive benefits.

Exhibit 8-1 Tranquility Health Care Center philosophy.

received final approval by the state inspection agency. The current target date is in mid-fall, about two months away.

The Center's Reputation

During the past few years, THCC has gained a reputation of the nursing home of choice in the city. This renown is attributed to its history of providing first class nursing care in a home-like atmosphere, for its exceptional cleanliness, and for living up to its slogan, "We're all about people." The center has maintained a 98 percent occupancy rate since 1985. People from throughout the city, county, and one neighboring state to the north seek placement in THCC for their family members.

---

1. Maintain a census of 98%
2. Increase the private pay census to 50%
3. Maintain or exceed an excess over expenses of $310,000
4. Maintain accounts receivable from private pay patients at 18 days.
5. Reduce employee accidents by 10%
6. Continue to receive superior rating by the Department of Health and Rehabilitative Services
7. Reduce employee turnover by 50%
8. Increase community relations programs
9. Remain union free
10. Reduce absenteeism by 25%
11. Reduce overtime by 50%

Exhibit 8-2 Tranquility Health Care Center corporate goals for fiscal year 1988.

The major referral sources are the two local hospitals and by word of mouth. THCC has prospered and its new, 36-bed wing nearing completion. The facility has received a superior rating from the Office of Licensure and Certification (OLC) for the past five years. A superior rating indicates that the center exceeds satisfactory standards for nursing home operation, and that it will receive a higher reimbursement rate from Medicaid than if it were rated less than superior. The OLC conducts an annual inspection and has been so impressed with the center that they have cited it as a model nursing home, and bring visitors to observe it. Representatives from the Health and Rehabilitative Services office survey Medicaid patients once a year. The Veterans Administration office conducts an annual inspection as well. The center has received recommendations for corrective action in only a few instances during the past five years. The organizational climate has been full of enthusiasm, high morale, and employees who seem to enjoy their work.

Organization and Administration

The organizational structure of THCC consists of the administrator and eight departments that comprise the management team (see Exhibit 8-3). Table 8-1 provides biographical information about the team members. At present there are 106 employees: 96 full-time

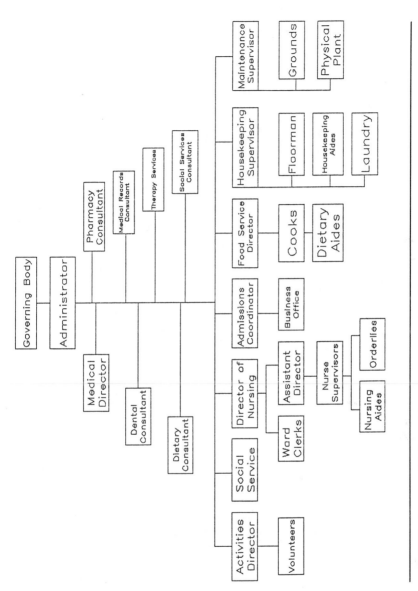

Exhibit 8-3 Tranquility Health Care Center organization chart.

Table 8-1 Management Team Biographical Data.

Team Member	Leadership Experience	Management Experience	Age	Education	Center Experience	Manager Meeting Participant
Administrator	10 yrs.	10 yrs.	67	2 yr. nursing	1.5 yrs.	Yes
Director of nursing	17 yrs.	11 yrs.	55	R.N. 3 years	6 yrs.	Yes
Assistant director of nursing	1.5 yrs.	5 yrs.	52	B.S.N.	21 mos.	Yes
Director of food services	13 yrs.	13 yrs.	40	High school	8 yrs.	Yes
Housekeeping/laundry	7.5 yrs.	-0-	33	1 yr. college	8 yrs.	Yes
Activities director	2 yrs.	4 yrs.	23	B.S. Ther. Rec	1 yr.	Yes
Maintenance supervisor	6 mos.	-0-	29	High school	6 mos.	Yes
Admissions/social service	8 yrs.	8 yrs.	33	B.A. Psychology	6 yrs.	Yes
Bookkeeper	3.5 yrs.	-0-	38	1 yr. college	3.5 yrs.	Yes
Ward clerk	14 yrs.	-0-	35	1 yr. Bookkeeping 1 yr. Business	8 yrs.	No
Supervisor/A-wing	1.5 yrs.	-0-	33	2 yr. R.N.	1.5 yrs.	No
Supervisor/B-wing	15 yrs.	10 yrs.	40	2 yr. R.N.	2.5 yrs.	No

and 10 part-time workers. The labor force is predominantly female, with only four male employees.

The Administrator

Sarah Ann Gustov is the administrator of THCC. The third administrator to occupy the leadership position under the present ownership, she is also the first female administrator in the center's history. Mrs. Gustov, a distinguished woman in her mid-sixties, is medium in stature and dresses conservatively with executive elegance. As the administrator for the past 18 months, she has proven to be very people-oriented. This attitude is reflected in her philosophy: ". . . to be sure my employees are functioning in a beneficial environment, which means their needs are met in all areas. This harmonious atmosphere shall reflect into nursing care, for ultimately we are all working for excellence in nursing care. When the needs of the employees and patients are met efficiently, a facility is profitable. When it is consistently profitable, all needs are being met."

The previous administrator, Mr. Burton, was not people-oriented and lacked diplomacy in handling the center's personnel. As a result, there was continuous conflict between him and his department managers, as well as dissention among the managers themselves. Mr. Burton had particular problems with the director of nursing services. The present administrator has attempted to create a more positive relationship with department heads. Mrs. Gustov often states, "I have impressed upon the employees that each department is as important as the other, and they must all work together on behalf of the residents."

Since Mrs. Gustov has been with the center, she succeeded in achieving her original goals including stabilizing relations among departments and between managers and the administrator, improving the center's cleanliness, and adding a feminine touch and a more decorative appearance to the environment. Live plants and bright and cheerful wallcoverings can be seen throughout the center. The underutilized day room was redecorated and converted to a very pleasant conference room with pictures, plants, and high quality furnishings since residents used a well furnished activity room for recreation purposes. The entire facility is immaculate, from the floors that are polished daily to the beautifully decorated resident rooms, sitting areas, and dining room. The atmosphere resembles a private residence filled with many family members rather than an institution.

Mrs. Gustov is an energetic, dignified, and compassionate person whose presence commands respect. She is often found walking down the halls, visiting residents, conferring with the staff, and ensuring that operations are smooth. She is justifiably proud that her facility is the highest rated in the community, and says that this rating is a testimony to the efforts of the dedicated department managers and their staffs. During the past six months, she has continued to make her daily rounds, but she says most of her time is spent making arrangements for the completion of the new wing. She is very concerned about the continuous construction delays because the facility loses revenue each day the opening is postponed. Mr. Harrison, the corporation's regional administrator who was the center's administrator for two years before Mr. Burton's tenure at THCC, is also concerned about the delay. He currently visits Mrs. Gustov at least once a month rather than the usual quarterly call.

On most days, Mrs. Gustov begins work at 8:00 A.M. and finishes at 5:00 P.M. Each morning at 8:30 she holds an administrative meeting for representatives from each department. They discuss issues from the previous day and prepare for the current day's activities. The meeting usually lasts from 15 to 20 minutes.

A monthly supervisory meeting is held during which staff are encouraged to voice their problems and suggestions for more efficient operation of the center. At this meeting a monthly budget report from the corporate office is distributed to the respective departments. The report, which details revenues and expenses, is sometimes discussed. The report does not include an analysis of units of service provided.

The Director of Nursing Services

Mrs. Gustov does not have an assistant administrator. The director of nursing services is a strong person who manages the center's largest labor force and assumes responsibility during the administrator's absence. Ingrid Stansbury is a registered nurse with 17 years of experience in nursing supervision. She has been employed at THCC for the past six years. She spent her first two years as a nursing supervisor, and was subsequently promoted to Director of Nursing Services. With a heavy northeastern accent and a good sense of humor, she maintains that she has to have broad shoulders since everyone blames nursing services for everything. Mrs. Stansbury is a dedicated nurse who is genuinely concerned that residents achieve their maximum potential. The THCC bookkeeper believes that Mrs.

Stansbury is directly responsible for the continued superior rating that the center enjoys. Active in professional organizations, she has served as president of the local chapter of the Directors of Long-Term Care Facilities for the past four years. She is honest, fair, and believes in leadership by example. Exhibiting a strong managerial style, she demands that high standards are met and maintained by her department. She is not bothered that some employees have told her that they do not like her. Being very outspoken and assertive, she has had occasional run-ins with Mrs. Gustov about the boundaries of authority.

The Nursing Department Structure and Staff

The departmental structure consists of an assistant director of nursing and two R.N. supervisors (one for the A wing and one for the B wing). Each wing has a staff consisting of one L.P.N. per shift and three to six nursing aides (Table 8-2).

Lisa Martin, the A wing supervisor, is a 33-year-old R.N. who has spent 1 and 1/2 years at the center. Ms. Martin, a former army nurse, is described by the director of nursing as a person who works well with doctors and can handle almost any emergency situation. At other times, however, she displays a negative attitude, appears unconcerned, and does not supervise the nurses' aides as closely as she should. On occasion she has said that she is sick of listening to her nurses' problems. She has also distanced herself from her staff by severely reprimanding aides in the presence of visitors.

Jessica Terry, the B wing supervisor, is a 40-year-old R.N. who has worked at the center for over two years. The director of nursing describes her as a qualified, energetic, and concerned nurse. Her strengths lie in patient and family relations. She is well liked by the residents and families and is considered to be kind and gentle. She communicates with the families, giving them feedback about their relatives. Ms. Terry has high performance expectations of the nurses and insists that they be efficient; on occasion, she has been accused of criticizing her staff excessively.

The THCC nursing staff can be readily identified by their uniforms which are neat, professional, and well coordinated. R.N.s and L.P.N.s wear white uniforms and shoes. The nurses' aides are dressed in white pants and blouse or dresses covered with maroon smocks. Every staff member wears a black and gold name tag, displays a warm smile, and is willing to lend a helping hand. The nursing station is also impressive. White formica with blue trim and

Table 8-2 Nursing service staffing pattern.

Shifts	R.N.s	L.P.N.s	Aides
A Wing			
7 A.M.–3 P.M.	1	1	6
3 A.M.–11 P.M.	1	1	5
11 A.M.–7 P.M.	1	0	3
B Wing			
7 A.M.–3 P.M.	1	1	6
3 A.M.–11 P.M.	1	1	5
11 A.M.–7 P.M.	1	0	3

brightly colored wallcoverings blend well with high quality furniture where residents often sit.

The director of nursing services has spent many hours making sure that resident care plans meet the standards of the OLC. She has held daily meetings for the past month with her assistant and the supervisors to update care plans so they will be current.

In addition to paying attention to care plans, Mrs. Stansbury has been frustrated by the high turnover rate among nursing assistants. While approximately 50 percent of the staff has been employed at the center for six to seven years and are very stable, the other half of the staff is unstable. Last year, the attrition rate for nursing assistants was 65 percent. In one week, four nurses' aides were hired. One worked for two days and one stayed for only one week before leaving. Nearly every month Mrs. Stansbury asks Nicky Bolden, the ward clerk and secretary, to place an ad in the newspaper for nursing assistants. She attributes the high turnover rate to the low salaries aides are paid at the center. They can obtain better salaries doing much cleaner work. There is a lack of public transportation in the area, and it is difficult for a person who only earns $4 an hour to get to work.

Mrs. Stansbury suggested, "We would be better off buying a couple of vans and running a shuttle service between the center and various points in the county so they could get to work." She also has had to discharge aides because of poor attitudes and performance.

Nursing assistants and nurses undergo a five-day orientation program upon being employed by the center. The focus of the first day of the program is on policies and procedures, and new employees spend the remaining four days on the unit with an experienced nurse. The corporate policy stipulates that the orientation period should not exceed five days. The director of nursing services believes that more time is needed to prepare some nurses to work independently. As a result, she has extended the orientation period for certain nurses despite the corporate policy.

Mrs. Stansbury is also concerned about the large amount of money spent for agency nurses which are used primarily on the 11 P.M. to 7 A.M. shift. Although unaware of last year's total expenditure in this category, she knows it is a "bundle." Some agencies charge as much as $15 per hour for an R.N.'s services.

A satisfaction survey has not been conducted for nursing services, nor is an employee exit interview system in operation. Mrs. Stansbury maintains that she is too busy to prepare any extra reports.

Dietary Services

Geraldine Cooper is the 40-year-old director of food services. She has been with the center for eight years and has had a total of 13 years of experience in dietary services. The dietary staff is dressed in white uniforms covered with gold smocks. Mrs. Cooper is dedicated to providing the residents a nutritious meal served at the proper temperature and in a timely manner. Lunch and dinner meals are available to employees for only $1.50 and generally, the food is considered good. Mrs. Cooper is respected by her staff which is very loyal to her. However, there has been some conflict in the past between the dietary department and other staff in the center. According to nursing service personnel, they have met with less than courteous and cooperative attitudes when they have visited the dietary department for lunch or inquired about services for patients.

Housekeeping

Phyllis Rogers, the housekeeping and laundry supervisor, is a 33-year-old woman with eight years of related experience. She has been with the facility since it was established. She is the motivating force behind Paul, the floor man, who keeps the floors shining constantly. Her staff is commended by the nursing service for their responsiveness to their needs for housekeeping services. Ms. Rogers visits the residents' rooms daily to be sure that they are kept in sparkling condition.

Activities

Diane Howard is the director of the activities department. She is 23-years-old and has been with the facility for one year. Although a competing nursing home tried to lure her away recently, she was persuaded to remain at THCC. Her responsibilities include planning and coordinating the many daily activities which give the residents enjoyment and structure (Exhibit 8-4).

As a result of an agreement with the state volunteer program, she has two full-time volunteers who assist Ms. Howard and the residents with their activities. Representatives from several church organizations visit the center frequently and provide church services, sing-alongs, and other entertainment. Sometimes residents attend what is known as a "love luncheon" at a local church. Athletic activities and bingo parties with ice cream and cake are also enjoyed at the center. Each resident is encouraged to participate in some activity. On Fridays, Ms. Howard coordinates a "Happy Hour" where certain residents visit the activities room to enjoy their favorite beverages. As a result of the director's work, the center is filled with laughter, songs, and music.

Bookkeeping and Payroll

Susan Peach, 38-years-old, has been with THCC for two years. With a friendly and outgoing personality, she generates a sense of sincerity, loyalty, and dedication to the center's operations. Ms. Peach is responsible for ensuring that the financial matters of the center and the residents are handled properly. Although she is preparing to take the nursing home administrator licensure examination in December, she devotes a great deal of time to her duties. Despite this, she has been frustrated for many months because of the many deadlines that the corporate office has imposed. She keeps the deadlines she sets for herself current on a monthly basis. Among other duties, she is responsible for monthly billing due by the 10th, a patient days and census report needed by the 15th, accounts receivable adjustments required by the 24th, and various end-of-the-month closings including accounts payable records and bank reconciliations that must be completed by the 30th of each month.

Ms. Peach's office is located in a very small room that leads into the reception area of the facility. Three desks are crammed into an office designed for one. Ms. Peach, the payroll clerk, and the switchboard operator occupy the room which also holds a copy machine used by all the staff. The bookkeeper and the payroll clerk agreed that the lack of space was a major problem.

Ms. Peach stated, "It is most frustrating to meet deadlines in an atmosphere where there are so many interruptions. My concentration is divided among my work, the people who come to use the copier, and the constant telephone calls and conversations of the receptionist and the switchboard operator. It causes me to make unnecessary mistakes. Mrs. Gustov promised that she would move me to a larger space in another part of the building, but she is too busy with getting the new wing opened."

Ms. Peach also expressed concern that the center may not be capturing all the charges that it should. She speculates that the lost charges could be as much as 50 percent of supplies used by the nursing service. However, she has such a heavy workload that she does not have time to visit the units to verify the charges submitted. She does, however, provide yearly inservice training to the nursing department on the charge sticker system which provides an account of expenses incurred. This system, used throughout the corporation, involves the use of white stickers that are placed on the charge sheet in the medical record of each resident. This charge sheet is then submitted to bookkeeping each month which uses this information to determine monthly charges for each resident. As a result of repeatedly receiving charge sheets that appeared to reflect less than the expected number of charge tickets, the bookkeeper decided to present the problem to the director of nursing. However, the director of nursing seemed to ignore the situation.

According to Ms. Peach, "All I got from her was that it was bookkeeping's fault, stemming from my obviously inaccurate records. She also chewed me out and reported me to the previous administrator for trying to get help from Nicky Bolden on the proper diagnosis coding needed to avoid rejection from Medicaid. She screamed at me and said that Nicky couldn't help me do my work. Everybody knows that Nicky has a lot of information about nursing home operations. She has been here since the place opened. She is smart and does lots of work and, in my opinion, is the only one who

SUNDAY	MONDAY	TUESDAY	WEDNESDAY
JUNE 1988			**1** 9:00 — Exercise (A/B) 10:00 — Lan. Skills (A/B) 11:00 — Learning Games (A/B) 1:30 — Cur. Events (A/B) 2:30 — Bingo (DR) 6:00 — Table Games/Cards (DR)
5 3:00 — Church (AR) 3:30 — Hymn Sing (AR) 6:00 — Bowling (AR)	**6** 9:00 — Exercise (A/B) 10:00 — Lan. Skills (A/B) 11:00 — Learning Games (A/B) 1:30 — Cur. Events (A/B) 2:30 — Life Skills (A/B) 6:00 — Cooking Class (AR)	**7** 9:00 — Exercise (A/B) 10:00 — Lan. Skills (A/B) 10:30 — Creative Preschool 11:00 — Learning Games (A/B) 1:30 — Cur. Events (A/B) 2:30 — Pet Visitation 2:30 — Life Skills (A/B) 6:00 — Crafts (AR)	**8** 9:00 — Exercise (A/B) 10:00 — Lan. Skills (A/B) 10:30 — .... (AR) ✓ 11:00 — Learning Games (A/B) 1:30 — Cur. Events (A/B) 2:30 — Bingo (DR) 6:00 — Table Games/Cards (DR)
12 3:00 — Church (AR) 3:30 — Hymn Sing (AR) 6:00 — Bowling (AR)	**13** 9:00 — Exercise (A/B) 10:00 — Lan. Skills (A/B) 11:00 — Learning Games (A/B) 11:00 — Love Luncheon 1:30 — Cur. Events (A/B) 2:30 — Life Skills (A/B) 2:30 — Sing-Along (AR) 6:00 — Reminiscence Group (AR)	**14** 9:00 — Exercise (A/B) 10:00 — Lan. Skills (A/B) 10:30 — Creative Preschool 11:00 — Learning Games (A/B) 1:30 — Cur. Events (A/B) 2:30 — Life Skills (A/B) 6:00 — Crafts (AR) Flag Day	**15** 9:00 — Exercise (A/B) 10:00 — Lan. Skills (A/B) 11:00 — Learning Games (A/B) 1:30 — Cur. Events (A/B) 2:30 — Birthday Party 6:00 — Table Games/Cards (DR)
19 3:00 — Church (AR) 3:30 — Hymn Sing (AR) 6:00 — Bowling (AR)	**20** 9:00 — Exercise (A/B) 10:00 — Lan. Skills (A/B) 11:00 — Learning Games (A/B) 1:30 — Cur. Events (A/B) 2:30 — Life Skills (A/B) 2:30 — Sing-Along (AR) 6:00 — Cooking Class (AR)	**21** 9:00 — Exercise (A/B) 10:00 — Lan. Skills (A/B) 10:30 — Creative Preschool 11:00 — Learning Games (A/B) 1:30 — Cur. Events (A/B) 2:30 — Life Skills (A/B) 6:00 — Crafts (AR)	**22** 9:00 — Exercise (A/B) 10:00 — Lan. Skills (A/B) 10:30 — .... (AR) ✓ 11:00 — Learning Games (A/B) 1:30 — Cur. Events (A/B) 2:30 — Bingo (A/B) 6:00 — Table Games/Cards (DR)
26 3:00 — Church (AR) 3:30 — Hymn Sing (AR) 6:00 — Bowling (AR)	**27** 9:00 — Exercise (A/B) 10:00 — Lan. Skills (A/B) 11:00 — Learning Games (A/B) 1:30 — Cur. Events (A/B) 2:30 — Life Skills (A/B) 2:30 — Sing-Along (AR) 6:00 — Cooking Class (AR)	**28** 9:00 — Exercise (A/B) 10:00 — Lan. Skills (A/B) 10:00 — Spelling Bee 10:30 — Creative Preschool 11:00 — Learning Games (A/B) 1:30 — Cur. Events (A/B) 2:30 — Life Skills (A/B) 6:00 — Crafts (AR)	**29** 9:00 — Exercise (A/B) 10:00 — Lan. Skills (A/B) 10:30 — .... (AR) ✓ 11:00 — Learning Games (A/B) 1:30 — Cur. Events (A/B) 2:30 — Bingo (A/B) 6:00 — Table Games/Cards (DR)

Exhibit 8-4 Calendar of resident activities and events.

THURSDAY	FRIDAY	SATURDAY
2 9:00 — Exercise (A/B) 10:00 — Lan. Skills (A/B) 11:00 — Learning Games (A/B) 11:00 — Rev. ⋯ (AR) ✓ 1:30 — Cur. Events (A/B) 2:30 — Life Skills (A/B) 3:00 — Happy Hour Visit 6:00 — Senior Sports (AR)	**3** 9:00 — Exercise (A/B) 10:00 — Lan. Skills (A/B) 11:00 — Lunch Trip 11:00 — Learning Games (A/B) 1:30 — Cur. Events (A/B) 2:30 — Bingo (DR) 6:00 — Table Games/Cards (DR)	**4** 10:00 — Track Team (AR) 10:30 — One on One Visits 1:30 — Cur. Events (AR) 2:00 — Videos (CR)
9 9:00 — Exercise (A/B) 10:00 — Lan. Skills (A/B) 11:00 — Learning Games (A/B) 11:00 — Rev. ⋯ (AR) ✓ 1:30 — Cur. Events (A/B) 2:30 — Life Skills (A/B) 6:00 — Senior Sports (AR)	**10** 9:00 — Exercise (A/B) 10:00 — Lan. Skills (A/B) 10:30 — Communion 11:00 — Learning Games (A/B) 1:30 — Cur. Events (A/B) 2:30 — Life Skills (A/B) 2:30 — Bingo (DR) 6:00 — Table Games/Cards (DR) **"Lottery"**	**11** 10:00 — Track Team (AR) 10:30 — One on One Visits 1:30 — Cur. Events (AR) 2:00 — Videos (CR)
16 9:00 — Exercise (A/B) 10:00 — Lan. Skills (A/B) 11:00 — Learning Games (A/B) 11:00 — Rev. ⋯ (AR) ✓ 1:30 — Cur. Events (A/B) 2:30 — Life Skills (A/B) 3:00 — Happy Hour Visit 6:00 — Senior Sports (AR) 7:30 — Family Council (AR)	**17** 9:00 — Exercise (A/B) 10:00 — Lan. Skills (A/B) 10:30 — Junior Museum Visit 11:00 — Learning Games (A/B) 1:30 — Cur. Events (A/B) 2:30 — Life Skills (A/B) 2:30 — Bingo (DR) 6:00 — Table Games/Cards (DR)	**18** 10:00 — Track Team (AR) 10:30 — One on One Visits 1:30 — Cur. Events (AR) 2:00 — Videos (CR)
23 9:00 — Exercise (A/B) 10:00 — Lan. Skills (A/B) 11:00 — Learning Games (A/B) 11:00 — Rev. ⋯ (AR) ✓ 1:30 — Cur. Events (A/B) 2:30 — Life Skills (A/B) 3:00 — Happy Hour Visit 6:00 — Senior Sports (AR)	**24** 9:00 — Exercise (A/B) 10:00 — Lan. Skills (A/B) 10:30 — Resident Council 11:00 — Learning Games (A/B) 1:30 — Cur. Events (A/B) 2:30 — Life Skills (A/B) 2:30 — Bingo (DR) 6:00 — Table Games/Cards (DR) **"Lottery"**	**25** 10:00 — Track Team (AR) 10:30 — One on One Visits 1:30 — Cur. Events (AR) 2:00 — Videos (CR)
30 9:00 — Exercise (A/B) 10:00 — Lan. Skills (A/B) 11:00 — Learning Games (A/B) 11:00 — Rev. ⋯ (AR) ✓ 1:30 — Cur. Events (A/B) 2:30 — Life Skills (A/B) 3:00 — Happy Hour Visit 6:00 — Senior Sports (AR)	LOCATION KEY: A — A Wing B — B Wing AR — Activity Room CR — Conference Room DR — Dining Room	

Exhibit 8-4, continued.

approaches being indispensable around here. I don't think it's fair that she would not be allowed to help me do a better job."

The Problem of the Delayed Opening of the New Wing

The annual operating budget for THCC is $5,588,000, with a projected excess of revenue over expense of $310,000. Mrs. Gustov calculated that the center was losing at least $2,000 per day (based on the daily Medicaid reimbursement rate of $53 per patient day) due to the delay in opening the new beds. Efforts were made to hold the contractors monetarily responsible for each day the wing did not open.

The administrator was well aware that much of her time had been dedicated to preparing for the new wing. Department managers had devoted much of their time to the project as well. Both the housekeeping and building maintenance departments had worked overtime to meet deadlines only to have the deadlines postponed.

A Consultant Analyzes the Center

In view of the demands associated with the opening of the wing of the center, Mrs. Gustov was happy to grant the request of an academic consultant from a local university to study long-term care administration at THCC for the summer. His purpose was to rotate through the center's departments, interview key personnel, and review policies and procedures in an attempt to identify problems and opportunities to improve operations.

On June 20, three weeks after the consultant's arrival, he made a verbal report to Mrs. Gustov which identified several areas for improvement. The list included:

1. Complaints by nursing service about the periodic shortage of linens and towels needed for the residents' care;

2. Loose procedures for receiving goods from vendors;

3. Poor documentation of charges for services on the nursing units;

4. Food wastage; and

5. High turnover rate of nursing aides.

Additionally, it was reported that nursing services, dietary services, and the business office were all generally aware of the recurring problems of lost charges and wastage. There is no monitoring system to determine if solutions to such problems are effective after they have been implemented. Finally, because of the high turnover rate among nursing aides, the time and money devoted to training them are virtually wasted.

Mrs. Gustov had always believed in delegating authority for running departments and had felt confident that her managers could handle their responsibilities. She had suspected that the problems of lost charges and food waste might exist, but had not had time to explore the situations personally; she left it up to the department managers to run the departments efficiently. In an effort to reduce operating expenses, Mrs. Gustov decided to have the consultant conduct a study of lost charges in nursing services and food wastage to determine the magnitude of these problems.

The Studies

Nursing Services Lost Charges

To determine the extent of lost charges, a sample was chosen of a month of nursing charges that had been submitted to the bookkeeping office. Because of the standardized activities associated with caring for diabetic residents, the charges of this group were selected for study. Medical records for ten diabetic residents from June were randomly selected. This sample size represented 50 percent of the total diabetic population at the center at the time of the study. Five charts were selected randomly from the A wing of the center and five were selected from the B wing.

Each record was first reviewed to determine what the doctors' orders were for both glucometer testing and insulin administration. This was indicated by the signature of the nurse performing the service. The number of procedures ordered was compared to the number of charge stickers submitted to bookkeeping for billing purposes for glucometer tests and syringes.

Findings. A significant number of charges were lost for both glucometer tests and insulin syringes (Table 8-3). The data show that the lost charges for glucometer tests were more severe than for

Table 8-3 Summary of data collected on ten diabetic residents for month of June.

Total no. lost charges	
Glucometer tests	242
Insulin syringes used	320
Glucometer tests, A wing	219
Insulin syringes used, A wing	201
Glucometer tests, B wing	23
Syringes used, B wing	119
Charge for	
Glucometer test	$1.85
Insulin syringe	$ .50
Total lost charge	
Glucometer tests (242 x $1.85)	$447.70
Insulin syringes (320 x $.50)	$160.00
Both glucometer test and syringes	$607.70
Average charge lost per patient	
Glucometer	$ 44.77
Syringe	$ 16.00
Total average charge lost per patient	$ 60.77
Total charges lost,	
Projected for one year ($607.70 x 12)	$7,292.40
Total charges lost for 20 residents,	
Projected for one year	$14,584.80

insulin syringes and more losses occurred with the A wing residents than with the B wing residents.

Glucometer testing was generally performed by nurse aides. There was a total of 242 uncharged glucometer tests performed. At a rate of $1.85 for each test, this represents a loss of $447.70 for the ten residents during the one month period. This is an average monthly loss of $44.77 per resident.

Insulin injections were usually given by R.N.s. The total number of insulin syringes used, but not charged, was 320. At a charge of $.50 per needle, this represents a loss of $160.00 for the ten residents for one month. This is an average monthly loss of $16.00 per resident.

The total lost charges for both glucometer tests and insulin syringes for the ten residents was $607.70 for one month. This amounts to an annual loss of $7,292.40. Assuming that the same pattern holds for the other ten diabetic residents, the loss is twice as great. The projection for one year of the 20 diabetic patients represents a loss of $14,584.80.

In view of the fact that similar charge losses could be occurring with the care of the 100 other residents at the center, the potential for lost charges due to improper use of the system for capturing charges is significant and certainly suggests the need for change.

Food Service Distribution and Waste

The study of the food service distribution system involved observation of meals served to the residents at breakfast, lunch, and dinner. Observations were conducted once during breakfast and dinner and twice during the lunch period. In most instances, both dietary workers and nursing aides demonstrated speed and concern for feeding patients in a timely manner. In two instances, however, trays were taken from the delivery cart and left for more than five minutes before being served to the resident.

One observation showed that meals had not been prepared for two of the residents; they were simply overlooked. Meals were prepared and brought to the unit within ten minutes of the discovery.

The most noteworthy problem identified was that the nurse aides discarded meals. Three reasons were identified:

1. Meals were thrown away when the patient had died. In the cases observed, one resident passed away the previous day, and another patient had passed away three days earlier. Three meals a day were wasted for each of these deceased residents.

2. Meals were thrown away when the resident ate outside the center. During one observation two meals were discarded; during another observation five meals were thrown away. The dietary department had been notified that the residents would be away from the center at lunchtime, but the information was not delivered to the appropriate personnel.

3. On occasion, meals were sent to the floors for patients who had been discharged. During the observations, three meals were thrown away for this reason.

Previous studies have shown that the average cost to prepare a meal at the center is $1.80. Sixteen meals were thrown away in four randomly selected observations during a two-week period. The unnecessary expense totalled $28.80.

The food service report was presented to Mrs. Gustov on a Friday afternoon at the end of August. She began to wonder if she could provide salary increases to the center's employees in light of such inefficiencies. She was also concerned that if expenses were not properly accounted for, it could adversely affect the end-of-year Medicaid cost report which determines the amount the center is reimbursed for services. Although she was concerned about these oversights, she believed that the quality of care provided to the residents had not suffered.

After presenting the report, the consultant left and Mrs. Gustov sat at her desk, pencil in hand, pondering her course of action.

Part IV

Financial Planning

Introduction

This section focuses primarily on issues of financial planning, reimbursement, and budgeting. Implications of Medicaid and Medicare reimbursement for financial viability is a theme addressed in these and other cases in the book. Management of case mix, staffing patterns, quality of care assessment, and regulation are major forces influencing the financial status of these organizations.

The first case, "The Need for a Marketing and Financial Plan," involves the need for greater fund-raising efforts in an adult day care center for demented patients. Since client fees do not cover costs, the organization must examine several options for generating additional revenue. If these development efforts do not succeed, the Family Respite Center might have to consider budget cuts.

Southern State Community Long-Term Care operates through contractual services with many local vendors. This case discusses how the fees of this public organization should be established and how service provisions should be monitored.

The Community Nursing Agency case reveals a financial crisis due to denial of Medicare claims for home health care. The financial shortfall is so serious that it has repercussions throughout the organization.

Each of these cases involves financial decision making in the context of other aspects of organizational functioning. In fact, these are the most complex cases in the book; they are complicated by issues of management style, operational procedures, and strategic planning—the major topic areas addressed by the book.

Case 9

The Need for a Marketing and Financial Plan: The Family Respite Center[*]

Lin E. Noyes, Donna Lind Infeld, and Richard Wittenborn

Lin E. Noyes, R.N., M.S.N., is the director of the Family Respite Center, Falls Church, VA.

Donna Lind Infeld, Ph.D., is Associate Professor, Department of Health Services Administration, School of Government and Business Administration, The George Washington University.

Richard Wittenborn, M.D., is the medical director of the Family Respite Center, Falls Church, VA.

Alzheimer's Disease Victims and Adult Day Care

While 85 percent of adults 65 years of age and over retain their mental abilities throughout their lives, 15 percent suffer from progressive memory loss, intellectual impairment, and the inability to care for themselves (National Institutes of Health 1981). There are many causes of dementia; some of them can be treated or cured. However, most dementias are progressive and irreversible. Alz-

---

[*] This case was based on L.E. Noyes and R. Wittenborn. 1987. *The Family Respite Center: Day Care for the Demented.* Falls Church, VA: Family Respite Center, Inc., developed with support from the Office of Technology Assessment; *Family Respite Center, Inc. Financial Statements Years Ended June 30, 1986 and June 30, 1987;* and R. R. Aptekar. 1984. *Plan for Implementation of an Adult Respite Day Care Center.* McLean, VA: North Star Planning and Management.

heimer's disease accounts for about half of irreversible dementia (Alzheimer's Disease and Related Disorders Association [ADRDA] 1983). Memory is gradually impaired early in the illness. As the disease progresses, personality may change and depression may appear. Later, impairments in both language and/or motor abilities are common. Eventually Alzheimer's victims lose their ability to eat, dress, and walk independently. In addition to functional difficulties, behavior problems frequently occur during the disease. Victims may babble, wander, or become hostile and abusive, and eventually become incontinent.

Despite substantial recent research, there is currently no cure for Alzheimer's disease. Even if a cure were found in the near future, there would still be the problem of providing care and help in day-to-day living for over 1.5 million Americans.

Most of the care for Alzheimer's patients is provided by family members. Providing this care is an emotionally and financially taxing job. Whereas most families try to keep their loved ones at home, when all resources are exhausted, often the nursing home is the only option available.

Adult day care programs for victims of Alzheimer's disease and related disorders are relatively new models of care to help support families who want to keep their family member in the community. While these programs meet a real community need, the lack of stable financing is a threat to their ongoing operation. This case study describes the services provided by the Family Respite Center of Falls Church, Virginia. Despite its status as a role model of adult day care programs for the demented, the center needs to expand marketing efforts and to review financial plans to ensure long-term viability.

Community Demand for a Respite Center

There are approximately 56,000 adults over 65 years of age in the three jurisdictions which make up the area known as Northern Virginia: Fairfax County (28,000), Arlington County (18,000), and the city of Alexandria (10,000). Based on estimates of 5 percent of this age group being severely demented and 10 percent more being mildly or moderately impaired, as many as 8,400 older persons in Northern Virginia may need adult respite day care services for support of dementia.

There were four adult day care centers in operation prior to the development of the Family Respite Center. These four centers served 144 clients per day, slightly above their planned capacity of 135. However, these centers provided care to only a few Alzheimer's patients—those with mild to moderate levels of the disease—but not those whose problems were more severe.

History of the Family Respite Center

The Alzheimer's Disease and Related Disorders Association, Northern Virginia Chapter (ADRDA NOVA) is a local chapter of a national organization founded in 1981 to provide family support, community education, and research assistance regarding conditions that result in dementia (ADRDA 1981). Individual chapters also help families find appropriate support services. As a need for services is identified, the ADRDA NOVA works to fill in the gaps in care, thus easing the burden of caregiving. One gap identified was the need for day care for severely impaired victims of dementing illnesses.

The idea of the Family Respite Center began with a meeting of an ADRDA NOVA support group in 1981 at which family caregivers expressed a need for help in caring for their relatives. As these patients' disease progressed and their abilities to perform activities of daily living (ADLs) diminished, they were turned away from day care centers that they had been attending or were refused admission to centers as new participants. Without day care, families had three options: nursing homes, in-home sitters, or giving the care themselves. The high cost of nursing homes and in-home sitters and the desire to keep a relative at home created the need to have an affordable respite alternative in the community. Specifically, these families needed daytime care for patients with Alzheimer's disease who were incontinent, wandered, or had tendencies to be violent or disruptive.

A committee was appointed by the ADRDA NOVA Board to develop a plan to provide this service in the northern Virginia area. The committee investigated the community's need for such a service, types of programs to meet the need, and sources of funding.

About a year after the idea of respite care was first discussed, committee members visited several adult day care centers, two of which catered to the victims of Alzheimer's-type illnesses. The Harbor Area Adult Day Care Center in Costa Mesa, California had a significant impact on development of a philosophy and goals for the proposed center. In addition to giving families respite, the Harbor Area Center also benefited its participants by slowing their decline, improving their functioning, and increasing their life satisfaction (Sands 1984). Burke Rehabilitation Center in White Plains, New York provided guidance to committee members in interior design, furniture, and other physical plant needs (Panella 1983). After visiting these centers, the goals of the proposed respite center in Northern Virginia were expanded to include a therapeutic program for the participants in addition to relieving the burden of the family.

The next step was to hire a consultant to develop a detailed plan for what was to become the Family Respite Center. The plan was accepted by the board in 1983.

The site selected for the center was an unused portion of a parochial high school which was available for one year. It was decided that it would be easier to promote an operating program rather than an idea. Therefore, the space was renovated, with considerable help from community volunteers. The Family Respite Center became a nonprofit corporation four years ago and two months later, the center was opened to provide care three days a week. Full-time operation began within a year.

Once operation began, the search for a permanent location was restarted. The Chesterbrook Presbyterian Church in Falls Church, Virginia, was selected as the permanent site. It was close enough to the original location to honor the commitment to the initial clients. It was also closer to areas with large concentrations of elderly persons and rent was reasonable. In June, the year after opening, the center moved to its present location.

Initial Funding

A donation of $11,000 in 1983 from the Knights of Columbus provided crucial support for planning and initial start-up expenses for the center. The only other funding sources were individual donations to ADRDA NOVA earmarked for the center. In 1984, the Knights of Columbus gave an additional $5,000, and the Clark Charitable Trust made a donation of $50,000. A grant from the Northern Virginia business community gave the center credibility and exposure in the community. These start-up funds ensured solvency for one year and permitted the director and the board of directors to concentrate on quality care and the evolution of the program.

Licensing of the Center

The Family Respite Center was granted provisional 501(C)(3) status until next year when the fiscal records of the corporation will be reviewed by the Internal Revenue Service. This designation is critical for fund raising and provides credibility for the center in the community.

The Family Respite Center was licensed by the Department of Social Welfare of the Commonwealth of Virginia. To be licensed, the center was required to have a zoning permit, building inspection, health department inspection, and fire inspection. It encompasses a global review of the Center's facilities and activities. There were specific requirements about the number of clients, the amount of space, and the facilities that must be provided. Licensing of nonprofit day care centers in Virginia is voluntary; however, the center's board felt that licensure would raise the community standard for adult day care for the elderly.

Program Goals

The program goals of the Family Respite Center are to (1) provide a stimulating day care program of social, physical, and creative activities for elderly persons with Alzheimer's disease and related disorders within an accepting and supportive environment aimed at maximizing the potential of each individual; (2) provide respite and support for the members of the families caring for persons with Alzheimer's disease and related disorders; and (3) prevent premature or inappropriate institutionalization, i.e., to allow persons with Alzheimer's disease and related disorders to remain in their own homes for as long as possible.

Participants

The center is designed to care for all demented individuals whose families can bring them for services. To date, only moderately to severely demented participants tend to use the center.

The center has provided over 8,456 hours of service to over 100 clients since it opened its doors four years ago. Over 3,000 hours were provided last year. (See Table 9-1 for enrollment trends.) There appears to be an increase in the number of new clients who are in more advanced stages of dementia. This trend is reflected in

Table 9-1 Client service record for last year (ending June 30).

	Days opened	Clients served	Participant days	No. of clients/day	Projected no. clients/day
This year					
Jun	22	29	335	15.2	20
May	21	30	333	15.3	20
Apr	21	25	323	15.4	20
Mar	23	25	357	15.5	20
Feb	18	26	302	16.7	20
Jan	19	21	241	12.7	20
Last year					
Dec	18	24	274	15.2	20
Nov	19	26	305	16.1	20
Oct	21	27	386	18.4	20
Sep	21	26	341	16.2	20
Aug	21	28	346	16.5	20
Jul	22	30	401	18.2	20

Note:

Days opened: The number of days during the month for which the center was opened to participants.

Clients served: The number of different individuals served during the month.

Participant days: Basic unit of measuring service; one client came for one day of service.

Average number of clients per day: Participant days divided by days opened for a month.

Projected average number of clients per day: This number is a basis for budgeting week.

the amount of assistance they need with ADLs such as eating, toileting, and walking; all the clients need help communicating. Table 9-2 shows demographic characteristics of the participants served in the last four years.

Operations

The center operates six days a week, Monday through Saturday, from 7:30 A.M. to 5:30 P.M. weekdays and from 10:00 A.M. to 5:00 P.M. Saturdays. The hours accommodate caregivers who commute to work, and staff hours are staggered to allow for an eight-hour work day. The center has a schedule of planned activities that are chosen to meet the clients' needs for physical exercise, rest, entertainment, and communication. Staff members are aware of the individual client's mood and lucidity, and tailor activities to their changing needs. In an effort to improve their community living skills, the clients are complimented and reinforced for their participation in an activity no matter how tangential that involvement may be.

Table 9-2 Comparison of client demographic characteristics.

	3 yrs. ago	2 yrs. ago	Last year	This year
Admissions	34	33	33	37
Men	11	18	13	17
Women	23	15	20	20
Spouse caregiver	18	19	20	20
Child caregiver	12	9	10	15
Other caregiver	4	5	3	2
Age range	48-93	49-93	53-89	59-103
Mean age	73	74	72.2	76
Ambulatory	28	29	31	32
Nonambulatory	6	4	2	5
Discharges	19	20	25	31
Death	5	5	2	0
Nursing home	3	6	9	18
Adult home	2	1	2	2
Out of area	2	2	2	0
Other centers	0	3	2	2
Families	6	0	8	9
Center request	1	3	0	0
Avg. length of stay (months)	3.69	4.03	9.20	10.6
Avg. attendance (days/week)	3.15	2.80	3.10	3.75

Note:

Ambulatory: Physically able to walk safely alone.

Nonambulatory: Physically unable to walk safely alone. The Department of Social Services has determined center clients to be "nonambulatory" for licensing purposes.

Individuals who choose not to join in an activity are asked how they feel about it and why they choose not to participate.

Families report that after initial adjustment, clients are more alert at home, sleep better at night, and have fewer outbursts of rage or overly anxious behaviors. There is a moderately high absenteeism rate because clients are very frail and are often unable to come to the center because of illness.

Structure and routine provide security for the clients with Alzheimer's disease. For this reason, a daily schedule is maintained and although length of activities may vary, one event always follows the next for continuity. A typical schedule is included as Table 9-3. Rest periods are regularly integrated into the schedule. To increase

Table 9-3 Typical daily schedule at the Family Respite Center.

Time	Activity
A.M.	
7:30-9:30	Drop off for early arrivals; coffee and conversation
9:30-10:45	Arrivals by most participants; semi-structured activities, including current events discussion, breakfast, group music. Orientation to the day.
10:45-10:50	Walk, toilet
10:50-11:45	Art projects
11:45-11:50	Snack
11:50-12:50	Exercise
P.M.	
12:50-1:15	Group sessions: discussions, expressive therapy
1:15-1:30	Lunch
1:15-1:30	Toilet
1:30-2:30	Video, slides, arts and crafts
2:30-3:30	Music, arts and crafts
3:30-4:00	Snack
4:00-5:30	Departures, structured individual or small group activities.

the likelihood of their sleeping through the night, participants do not take naps during the day.

Programming

In the past, after a relative would be diagnosed as having Alzheimer's disease, the family was told to do the best they could and start looking for a nursing home. There were no therapeutic goals of care except medication for unacceptable behaviors. The Family Respite Center, being in the forefront of care and treatment for people with Alzheimer's disease, provides a therapeutic program using milieu therapy and expressive therapy.

Milieu Therapy. During the 1960s, the Institute of Gerontology at the University of Michigan applied the theory of therapeutic milieu (i.e., certain elements in the environment enhance a patient's ability to regain or maintain levels of function) to a group of older adults, many of whom were suffering significant cognitive decline (Boudreault 1975). Generally, milieu therapy involves a structured, sheltered, supportive environment where patients are given tasks within their abilities and are praised and supported for their successes and contributions to the group. The use of this therapy significantly improves the participants' life satisfaction which seems to benefit their overall emotional welfare.

Expressive Therapy. A unique component of the center's program is expressive therapy. Through art, music, and movement, participants have an opportunity to express themselves. Thoughts and feelings that have been walled in by increasing impairment are given an avenue of communication. Art works produced are a measure of the client's progress at the center. The clients also derive satisfaction and pleasure out of constructing something individually or contributing to the work of the group. Individual sessions including assessments of participants' functional abilities are held three to four hours per week.

Reality orientation is not used as a therapy at the center. Although clients are frequently oriented to their surroundings and circumstances, the emphasis is on their awareness of the immediate present, not necessarily current events or circumstances outside the center.

Restraints of any kind are considered "last measure" therapies and are only used when their absence would prevent an otherwise desirable participant from attending the center. "Chemical restraints" are used only during brief periods of hyperactivity or anxiety and their use is reviewed monthly and discontinued as soon as possible. Geri-chairs have been added recently to the center only for those individuals who would endanger themselves if they walked without supervision. They are not used to limit mobility or interaction with the environment.

Education/Support Services and Information and Referral

Other center services focus on education and support for families and community care providers. Daytime family support groups meet twice a month and are open to the community. In these groups, families gain strength and support from each other by sharing experiences, insights, and resources. The center also offers a four-week course designed to give families knowledge about Alzheimer's disease and to prepare them for hands-on caregiving.

In addition, visits to the center and community speaking engagements have helped to spread the word about Alzheimer's disease and respite care. The center received over 1,000 phone calls last year requesting free information on Alzheimer's disease or desiring help for Alzheimer's victims.

Administration

The Board of Directors

The initial board of seven directors for the Center consisted of members of the ADRDA NOVA Planning Committee. The bylaws called for a board of between seven and 14 members, three of whom would be members of the ADRDA NOVA Board of Directors. The interlocking directorate ensures that the people in the community have access to all levels of the center, and that a number of members of the board have a personal commitment to patients with Alzheimer's disease. Some board members were selected from outside the ADRDA chapter in order to maintain the independence of the two organizations and to preserve their somewhat divergent purposes.

The board was designed to be a working board with members recruited to assist with specific needs, such as financial planning, fund raising, or marketing. A provision was made for a second, honorary board to include individuals who have an interest in the center and were willing to support it but could not make the significant time commitment required of full board members.

Board meetings are held quarterly, although extra meetings have occurred monthly to meet the needs of the rapid development of the center. There is a provision in the bylaws for telephone polling of the board, which ensures members' active involvement in major decisions. The board of directors sets policy for the center's operation, approves a yearly budget, acts on applications for scholarships, and takes an active role in raising money for the center. The board has several subcommittees to address specific tasks such as fund-raising campaigns, planning renovations of the center facilities, and marketing.

The medical director, a local neurologist, is on the board and advises the center director regarding participant behaviors and possible effects of medications. The medical director also approves health procedures such as the recent implementation of universal precautions to reduce the possible spread of infectious diseases.

Staff of the Center

The center has a paid staff consisting of a director, assistant director, six program assistants, and an art therapist. The ratio of staff to clients is at least one-to-five and has recently reached one-to-three.

The director was responsible for establishing day-to-day policies and procedures during the start-up of the center, and integrating the center with other services in the community. The director also has ongoing responsibility for an outreach program that involves generating talks within the community which raise the level of interest in and understanding of Alzheimer's disease and adult day care services. The director is also responsible for staffing, reviewing admissions and discharges, overseeing overall functioning, and is an *exofficio* member of the board.

Among the important qualifications for all of the staff are genuine concern for the participants and the ability to perceive them as parts of a larger family and community who are served by the Family Respite Center. They are dedicated and exhibit a willingness to learn and adapt to the wide range of client behavior encountered at the center. Staff turnover is low. Whereas staff are not particularly well paid, salaries are slightly higher than in local nursing homes. The small size and flexible nature of the organization seem to enhance staff commitment.

Volunteers

Volunteers provide innumerable hours of direct services to participants and help with other center activities. Volunteer involvement increases the personal attention each client receives and significantly supplements staff efforts. Volunteers are especially valuable during lunch time, arts and crafts, exercise, singing; they do office work, transport clients to beauty shops, shopping, and other special program events.

Budgeting and Revenues

The initial budget for the center was based on an expectation of 20 participants per day. Given 20 days of service per month, there would be 400 participant days of service per month. Based on an annual budget of $122,923 (Table 9-4), which is $10,244 per month, the total cost per participant per day is slightly more than $20. A daily fee of $22.80 was calculated to allow the center to roughly break even at capacity.

Most expenditures are directly related to program services. As with most service organizations, salaries are the largest expense. Table 9-5 details the center's financial situation.

No patient is turned away from the center for lack of funds and therefore an active scholarship program is supported by the community to provide either partial or complete assistance. Because of this subsidy, the center needs continuing community support. The center does not plan to cover all expenses from client fees, yet fees have become increasingly important as the patient population escalates.

Discussion

The Family Respite Center has served participants for over four years and has successfully achieved its primary goal of providing respite to the families of demented adults in the late stages of their disease. Severely demented individuals now have a less costly alternative to nursing home care. If the concept of an independent center is not viable for financial reasons, perhaps features in its programming can be extracted and applied in other settings. Whether or not this center presents a successful alternative as an independent service, replicable by others, remains a question.

The center's presence in the community has had an effect beyond the provision of day care for participants. At least one other area day care center has recently developed a special program for demented patients.

The center also has become an educational site for professionals, educators, researchers, and families to observe and learn about caregiving for demented patients. Local nursing home administrators have also consulted the center about opening special Alzheimer's units. In addition, many families have participated in classes for caregivers and support groups. It is clear from the interest

Table 9-4 Operating budget.*

Expenses	Annual Expense
Direct Labor	
Director	$ 30,000
Assistant director	19,000
Program assistants (2 @ $12,000/yr)	24,000
General assistant (1/2 time @ $12,000/yr)	6,000
Subtotal	79,000
Fringe benefits @ 10%	7,900
Payroll taxes	5,348
Total direct labor	$ 92,248
Other direct costs	
Telephone	1,200
Office supplies (consumable)	300
Meal preparation service ($2/meal)	12,000
Insurance	3,000
Accounting	500
Attorney	1,000
Rent, utilities and maintenance	9,375
Activity and participant consumables	
(@ .25/part./day)	1,500
Printing and postage	1,200
Publicity	600
Total other direct costs	$ 30,675
Total expenses	$122,923

*Based on an average daily attendance of 20 participants.

expressed about the center that it offers services different from other day care centers and that it is meeting a need for practical information on taking care of Alzheimer's victims.

While attaining program goals, the center has not reached its business goal of providing 20 patient days of care, five days a week. The average cost per day is higher than $22.80 and therefore the budget must be supplemented by ongoing fund raising. Budget projections show that $22.80 is an achievable goal, but the viability of the center, as a business, hinges on its running at full capacity.

There are several possible reasons for low utilization. First, adult day care, and specifically adult day care for dementia patients, is a relatively new concept and is only slowly gaining acceptance as an

Table 9-5 The Family Respite Center financial status report.

**Statement of Assets and Liabilities–Cash Basis
as of June 30**

	2 years ago	Last year
Assets		
Current assets		
Cash	$21,249	$14,228
Short-term investments	21,210[a]	29,128
Receivable from ADRDA	1,238	1,133
Hair Care Receivable	98	224
Total current assets	43,795	44,713
Property and equipment		
Donated property	4,800[b]	4,800
Furniture and office equipment	3,051	3,152
Less accumulated depreciation	(292)	(918)
Total property and equipment	7,559	7,034
Other assets		
Leasehold improvements (net of accumulated Amortization of $3,974)	6,159	4,113
Long-Term Investments	–	3,791[c]
Total other assets	$57,513	$59,651
Liabilities and fund balances		
Liabilities		
Payroll Taxes Payable	1,728	1,635
Other Liabilities	2	0
Total liabilities	1,730	1,635
Fund balances		
Current Unrestricted Fund	55,783	58,016
Total fund balances	55,783	58,016
Total liabilities and fund balances	$ 57,513	$59,651

---

[a] Interest-bearing mutual fund.

[b] Donated property includes a baby grand piano ($3,000) and a refrigerator ($1,800).

[c] 100 shares of stock.

Table 9-5, continued.

**Statement of Revenue, Expenses, and Fund Balances–Cash Basis
as of June 30**

	2 Yrs Ago	Last Year
Revenue		
Donations		
Grants and large donations	$18,950	$20,763[d]
Scholarship donations	1,500	17,294
Memorial donations	2,764	735
General donations	13,737	27,010
Designated donations	2,500[e]	0
Art therapy donations	8,066	0
Total donations	47,517	65,802
Other revenue		
Client fees	36,630	47,191
Conference fees	5,036	562
Interest and dividends	2,209	947
Other income	716	159
Total other revenue	44,591	48,859
Total revenue	92,108	114,661
Expenses		
Program services		
Amortization	1,542	1,685
Conference	5,725	380
Consumables	1,465	1,472
Consulting fees	0	25
Depreciations	218	523
Food	5,641	7,102
Inservices	61	144
Insurance	1,014	2,404
Other program service expenses	546	715
Open house expenses	979	0
Rent	4,400	5,200[f]
Printing, postage and publicity	671	663
Salaries	36,141	63,610
Taxes-payroll	3,200	5,618
Telephone	505	695
Total program services expense	$62,108	$90,236

[d] Scholarships have resulted in lost income of $15,034 two years ago and $24,482 last year.

[e] Designated for internal improvements.

[f] Rental commitments for 1988: $6,000; 1980: $6,000.

Table 9-5, continued.

Statement of Revenue, Expenses, and Fund Balances–Cash Basis

Supporting services		
General administration		
Amortization expense	385	362
Depreciations	24	51
Insurance	1,014	303
Legal and accounting	906	780
Office expense	1,599	1,894
Rent	1,100	975
Salaries	13,175	8,808
Taxes-payroll	1,163	713
Total general administration expenses	19,366	13,886
Fund raising	8,352	8,306
Total supporting services expenses	27,718	22,192
Total expenses	89,826	112,428
Excess of revenue over expenses	2,282	2,233
Beginning fund balances	53,501	55,783
Ending fund balances	$55,783	$58,016

alternative to nursing home care. In addition, acceptance of this type of center by health professionals and psychosocial professionals in the community is a slow process. The view of the center as filling in the gap between established day care centers and institutions has not been an easy concept to convey.

Another reason for low utilization is that whereas families who use the center are knowledgeable about Alzheimer's-type illnesses, are aware of their options for care, and understand the benefits of the program, this awareness is not widespread within the community. Further, the center has traditionally offered only basic services in an attempt to reach a cost-effective status where costs are covered by revenue. For example, no transportation or other services that are offered by other centers are provided. Families may perceive these extras to be desirable for their loved ones and therefore clients who may be appropriately served by the Family Respite Center go to other centers.

Conclusion

The case of the Family Respite Center introduces several important management problems. These include:

1. What kind of financial plan and/or fund raising effort is needed for the Family Respite Center?

2. What kind of marketing effort is appropriate for this type of organization?

3. Are other management or program changes indicated by the case?

References

Alzheimer's Disease and Related Disorders Association, Inc. 1981. *A national association to combat this silent epidemic.* Chicago: Alzheimer's Disease and Related Disorders Association.

Alzheimer's Disease and Related Disorders Association, Inc. 1983. *Fact sheet on Alzheimer's disease.* Chicago: Alzheimer's Disease and Related Disorders Association.

Boudreault, M.F. 1975. *To live with dignity: A report of a project with the frail and withdrawn.* Ann Arbor: Institute of Gerontology.

National Institutes of Health. 1981. *The Dementias–Hope through research.* Bethesda, MD: National Institutes of Health.

Panella, J., and H. Fletcher. 1983. *Day care for dementia. A manual of instruction for developing a program.* White Plains, NY: The Burke Rehabilitation Center, Dementia Research Service.

Sands, D. 1983. *Opening a day care center for persons with Alzheimer's disease and related disorders.* Costa Mesa, CA: Harbor Area Adult Day Care Center.

Sands, D. 1984. The harbor area adult day care center: A model program. *Pride Journal of Long-Term Care* 3(4):44–50.

Case 10

The Price is Right?: Community Long-Term Care*

William R. Koprowski

William R. Koprowski, Ph.D., CMA, NHA is Assistant Professor, College of Health Related Professions, Medical University of South Carolina.

Among the many areas with potential for cost reductions in the provision of long-term care services is the management of provider contracts. Although this area is rarely overlooked, actions to reduce expenditures are not often implemented. Concerns about internal operational efficiencies often obscure the cost savings that could be generated by focusing on the management of provider relationships. The Southern State Community Long-Term Care program began to explore potential approaches to reducing the costs of community long-term care services.

Overview

Southern State Community Long-Term Care (CLTC) serves elderly or disabled adults who want to live at home, need assistance to do so, and are eligible for nursing home admission under Medicaid. Last year in Southern State, well over 12,000 patients benefited from the program at a cost of approximately $8,000 per

---

* Fictitious names of both the organization and individuals are used to ensure anonymity. Facts and issues were modified to enhance teaching value.

person; considerably less than the cost of traditional nursing home care. The past success of the program and its potential for future cost containment, in light of the ever-increasing demand for Medicaid nursing home beds, has resulted in significant support for the program from the state and has solidified its position as a government provider of health services.

Because Medicaid eligibility is a prerequisite for CLTC participation, there has been little competition from private providers for the CLTC patient. In fact, there is tacit support for the program from local nursing home administrators since CLTC serves those people who otherwise would be "non-paying" nursing home patients.

CLTC has recently received a waiver for the care and treatment of AIDS patients in the state. It is expected that this expanded mission will necessitate a substantial increase in funding and staff.

CLTC is a division of the Southern State Health Services Financing Commission. The program started in 1978 as a Health Care Financing Administration, Research and Demonstration Project. The objective of the project was to assess the feasibility of caring for nursing home eligible patients who preferred to live at home. Since then, the program evolved into an integral part of the health care continuum in Southern State. Motivating this evolution were impressive facts from the demonstration project. Implementation of the Community Long-Term Care program resulted in reductions in Medicaid nursing home admissions by 16 percent and institutional patient days by an average of 37 percent.

While some programmatic attempts at community-based long-term care have not been financially viable, CLTC owes its success to the a priori dollar limit of services available to a client. As long as the cost of providing services in the home is less costly than the cost of institutional care, clients can select the alternative that meets their needs and preferences best. Once the cost exceeds that of institutional care; they must choose the nursing home alternative.

Services available to CLTC patients include personal care aide services; home delivered meals; medical day care; medical social services; and physical, speech, and occupational therapies. An integral component of the program and the major distinguishing feature of CLTC from traditional home health resources is case management. CLTC does not provide services directly to the client, but rather develops a care plan for each client which identifies individual needs and services necessary to meet these needs. CLTC then contracts for these services from a wide variety of providers, both individuals and large agencies, across the states. The care plan is developed with input from the patient, family, physician, and service providers.

Program elements consist of:

1. **Assessment.** Medical, social, environmental, and financial needs are evaluated to determine if the individual meets nursing home level of care criteria and is financially eligible for and interested in the community long-term care option.

2. **Case Management.** A care plan is developed to identify the most cost effective manner of providing services to meet the individual's needs.

3. **Monitoring.** Clients are monitored to ensure that services meet their needs and that any status changes are reflected in their plans of care.

Organization of the Program

A division of the Health Services Financing Commission, CLTC is comprised of three departments: 1) Field Management, 2) Professional Support Services, and 3) Program Development (see Exhibit 10-1). These departments are staffed by individuals with a masters' degree and over ten years of administrative experience.

The head of Field Management controls ten area offices through which day-to-day program operations are conducted. The head of Support Services has responsibility for a variety of staff activities including service authorization, provider relations, training, and quality assurance. Coordinators under her control provide technical support directly to Area Managers and their subordinates in the area offices. For example, although the billing clerk reports through the area manager to the head of Field Management, technical questions about billing errors are directed to the coordinator of Provider Relations, who reports to the head of Support Services.

The ten area managers reporting to the head of Field Management are employees of the Health and Human Services Financing Commission (as are other central office staff). They are specifically responsible for overseeing the level of care determinations, service authorizations, and case management. In addition to the area manager, the staff at each office includes one or more service

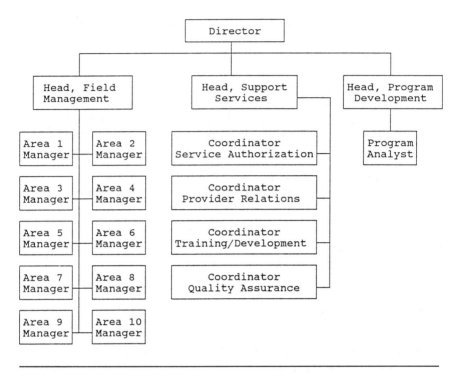

Exhibit 10-1 Community long-term care organization chart.

managers (depending on the size of the area office), either nurses or social workers, a secretary, a data clerk, and a billing clerk (Exhibit 10-2).

Except for area managers, area office staff are employees of the Department of Health and Environmental Control, a department with similar stature and organizational standing as the Health and Human Services Financing Commission.

Program Changes are Suggested

Brad Sherman, Coordinator of Provider Relations, received the following memorandum (through his immediate superior, the head of Support Services) from Dr. Davis, the Director.

Memorandum

Dear Brad,

In a conversation I had recently with a professor and friend, Roberta Lee, Ph.D., the topic of pricing provider services came up. She suggested that with our knowledge of *our* providers' costs we should consider variable pricing as a means for driving the best bargain for contract services. When I told her that I honestly wasn't quite sure what she was driving at, she offered to meet with you (I told her you were our resident expert in financial matters).

I am also concerned about the integrity of our billing system. How effective is our policy for monitoring the appropriateness of our payment for services. Are we paying for something the patient is not getting? I am truly concerned that we do our utmost to ensure we avoid this potentially embarrassing situation. Please discuss these matters with Dr. Lee and see if this variable pricing method can be of any benefit to us and whether we can do anything to improve our billing system.

I would like you to prepare a position paper on these two points. I need to know where we stand and what our options are. Although I am particularly interested in any cost savings that could be generated, I am equally concerned that any recommendations be "implementable" within the current organizational context. Remember, our financial wherewithall is limited, so avoid additional costs.

I'd appreciate a response at the beginning of next week.

Thanks,

J. Davis, M.D.

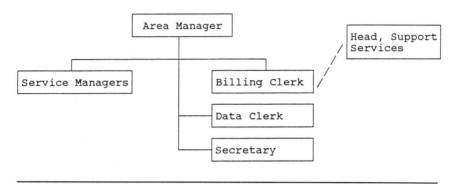

Exhibit 10-2 Area office organization chart.

Pricing Methodologies

Fortunately, Roberta could meet with Brad the following day. She opened the discussion by asking Brad to explain precisely how prices are determined for individual contract services. Brad suggested they look at Personal Care Aide service as an example since this accounts for the largest share of the Department's costs. Roberta agreed. Brad gave her the following information extracted from the most recent provider cost survey and explained that on an annual basis participating providers submit their cost information to the Department, which in turn, calculates average costs to be used for the service prices of the coming year (Table 10-1).

Roberta then asked Brad how he thought the system was working and what changes he would make if he had the authority. He stated that he was not totally certain that any major changes were needed. Although he was somewhat concerned that provider costs had increased at an annual rate of approximately 10 percent (much higher than inflation would suggest) for the past three years, he was more concerned that if the going rate were not paid, there might be difficulty in locating providers in the rural areas of the state. Moreover, if the price CLTC paid providers for their services was less than the costs they incurred to provide the services, how could they stay in business? Even if prices were somewhat inflated, the providers were happy with the present system. Moreover, a study conducted earlier in the year reported that clients, for the most part, were extremely pleased with the service they received. A small

Table 10-1 Provider cost survey information (Personal Care Aide).

	Per Visit Range	
Wage rate	$4.70 –	$5.00
Supplies	.70 –	.80
Travel	1.90 –	2.00
Depreciation (allocated fixed cost)	.20 –	1.70
Administrative (allocated fixed cost)	2.00 –	4.00
Total	$9.50 –	$13.50
Average		$11.50

minority were not happy with the recurring change in service providers, but they endorsed the CLTC program overall and were particularly positive about interaction with their case managers.

Perusing the survey data, Roberta quickly noted there was very little variance among certain categories while others differed considerably. She told Brad to review the fixed costs and informed him that considerable savings could be generated if service pricing approximated more nearly the variable cost of providing service, at least in the short run (although she did not specify an exact level). "Variable pricing is the answer," she exclaimed.

Brad still was not certain how prices could be reduced to less than their full cost and still provide the incentive necessary for providers to offer services. He explained to Roberta that the number of providers they use had grown to almost unmanageable limits. He estimated that there were over 200 providers with whom he had to work. When Roberta asked how providers were selected, Brad gave her the following information extracted from the department's policies and procedures manual.

A. All potential providers are subject to a pre-contract review. If the provider meets the requisite criteria (e.g. appropriate licensure and liability insurance), it is certified and a contract, on an annual basis, is initiated by the central office.

B. Once certified, providers are placed on the provider list organized and managed by geographic area

offices, and, if the patient has no provider preference, selected when needed.

C. Should a provider be incapable of or opt not to
provide the requested services, the next provider on
the list will be offered the opportunity.

The Billing System

Brad shared Dr. Davis's second concern about the billing system,
particularly since financial belt-tightening had curtailed the auditing
capabilities of the department. He noted, however, that one of the
conditions of the contract required providers to maintain financial
records for periodic auditing by the Medicaid Agency.

To demonstrate the billing process to Roberta, Brad prepared
the diagram as shown in Exhibit 10-3. He explained that the service
manager at the area office determines the individual's plan of care,
specifically noting the types, quantities and dates of services to be
performed. The service manager forwards this information to the
provider by telephone and concurrently sends copies to the billing
clerk.

The provider performs the service, has the patient or family
acknowledge the services rendered, and then submits a bill to the
billing clerk at the area office. The billing clerk compares the billed
services with the scheduled (requested) services and then forwards
the bill to the central office. The central office mails a check directly
to the provider. Bills are submitted any time from a week to a
month following service provision.

It has been reported that the area office is billed for services
that were not delivered even though they were on the calendar. A
retroactive adjustment must consequently be initiated. To ensure
that patients are getting the services for which the providers are
billing, service managers routinely check with patients and families.
Patients are quick to bring missed visits to the attention of the
service manager.

Brad added that he was amazed the system worked as well as it
did given the variety of reporting relationships and employers
involved in the program. After hearing this review of the system,
Roberta suggested that the department consider electronic billing.
Brad told her that he had considered this option (the computer
capability existed), but was not sure the benefits would outweigh the
costs. Although movement from manual to electronic billing could

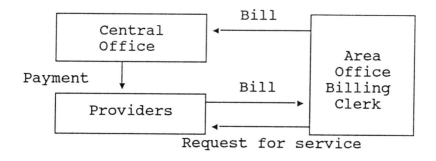

Exhibit 10-3 Billing process diagram.

potentially reduce administrative costs, he was not sure he wanted to expedite the department's payables (previous estimates suggested that days in accounts payable would decrease dramatically). Roberta suggested he look into it in more detail.

After his conversation with Roberta, and with much effort, Brad adopted the following outline for his position paper.

    A.   The Present Pricing Methodology
        1. Advantages
        2. Disadvantages

    B.   The Variable Pricing Methodology
        1. Advantages
        2. Disadvantages

    C.   Other Approaches
        1. Advantages
        2. Disadvantages

    D.   Billing System Problems

    E.   Organizational Impediments

    F.   Recommendations
        1. Pricing
        2. Billing

Now all that was left was to fill in the blanks—first thing tomorrow!

Case 11

Financial Crisis at the Community Nursing Agency[*]

Diane Brannon

Diane Brannon, Ph.D., is Assistant Professor of Health Planning and Administration, College of Health and Human Development, The Pennsylvania State University.

If you had asked staff at the Community Nursing Agency (CNA) early this summer, they would have told you things were really changing. What most staff did not yet know was that a fiscal crisis was brewing. A home health system that, in its 19-year history, had grown steadily both in services volume and complexity, was falling short of its projected service levels for the year, and facing a revenue shortfall. Both environmental and internal factors had contributed to the current situation. The case that follows describes the events and administrative activities as they developed during the summer.

A Brief History of the CNA

The Community Nursing Agency began operations in 1968 out of a county nursing home in western Pennsylvania. Initial funding was received from the Office of Economic Opportunity, the United Way, private contributors, and county government. A merger with the "county-seat" city nursing service was concluded and Medicare/Medicaid certification followed in 1969.

---

[*] Fictitious names of both the organization and individuals are used to ensure anonymity.

As the sole community provider of home health services, the agency grew throughout the 1970s in response to new opportunities. At the time of certification, new services were added to complement the home nursing therapies provided. These new services included homemaker and home health aide services, respiratory; occupational, and physical therapies; nutrition counseling; and social services. Hospice home care and volunteer programs were added as federal, state, and local funding sources became available. In 1973, a Maternal–Child Health Program received its first state funding and in 1977 a Women, Infants and Children's Supplemental Food Program was added. Following the closure of a nearby state hospital for the mentally ill, the agency began receiving state funding for community-based case management of de-institutionalized mentally ill and retarded individuals. Since 1980, contracts with the Area Agency on Aging enabled the agency to provide homemaker and/or chore services to support elderly clients remaining in their own home. The breadth of the agency's service mission is reflected in its mission and goal statement.

Mission and Goal Statement

Mission

The Community Nursing Agency's mission is to contribute to the overall well-being of the people in our community by facilitating the provision of quality in-home and community-based health care services that are affordable and available to all those in need.

Goals

1. To provide a broad range of health care services to help people attain their maximum state of health and comfort in their home environment.

2. To provide supportive care services and resources to assist families and individuals to live independently in their own community.

3. To develop financial resources that will support the mission of the agency and ensure its ability to meet the needs of the community.

4. To provide for the health-related resource needs of patients, families, agency staff, and allied health organizations.

In addition to its steady growth in services and programs, the Community Nursing Agency expanded geographically. In response to requests from physician groups and community leaders, branch offices were opened in four neighboring counties since 1972. Each branch office had a local advisory board and a manager who reported to central administration. Two years ago, the agency employed over 500 staff in these nine offices within the five counties (See Table 11-1 for program statistics). Fiscally, the agency had grown conservatively under the guidance of its community-based board of directors, and currently holds fixed assets of more than $300,000 including its central office building. The annual operating budget has exceeded $6,000,000 for several years.

Internal Factors

Last January, an organizational restructuring process culminated in a new corporate structure. The agency's board had embarked on this process at the request of the executive director in order to maximize funding resources and position the agency for future development. The new structure included a parent company (the Community Nursing Agency [CNA] Affiliates) and four subsidiaries (Exhibits 11-1 and 11-2). The Visiting Nurse Association became one subsidiary and assumed responsibility for the home health program. A new nonprofit subsidiary, Community Services (CS), was created to deliver supportive services such as private duty nursing, homemaker services, and other nonmedical programs. The third subsidiary was the Community Nursing Agency Foundation and the fourth a new for-profit company, Health Resources, which would allow CNA the flexibility of pursuing related ventures in the emerging home care market. Former assistant directors and administrators became chief operating officers and vice presidents' respectively; the executive director became the chief executive officer.

The change in structure reflected a move toward increased centralization and away from a relatively loose conglomerate of county agencies. While the process of reorganization was accomplished without open conflict, underlying tensions regarding the increased centralization of resources surfaced occasionally. For

Table 11-1 Community Nursing Service program statistics.

Staff

Administrators	6	Homemaker/home aides	260
Department and program managers	21	Nutritionists and nutrition aids	9
Registered nurses	125	Therapeutic activity workers	5
LPNs	25	Certified occupational Therapy assistants	3
Social workers	5	Business office	6
Physical therapists	12	Secretarial/clerical	32
Occupational therapists	2	Supportive services	24
Speech therapists	6	Total Agency Staff	553
Additional contract personnel	12		

Professional Visits

Home care*	176,822
Maternal-child–nursing, social service, homemaker/home health aide, and chore	2,749
Community support–nursing, therapies, homemaker/home health aide, chore, partial care, mental health social rehabilitation program	55,591
Hospice*	6,619
WIC enrollment	3,599
Total visits	241,781
Total individuals served	10,310

*Includes nursing, therapies (physical therapy, occupational therapy, speech therapy), medical social services, homemaker/home health aide, chore, companion, respite, attendant

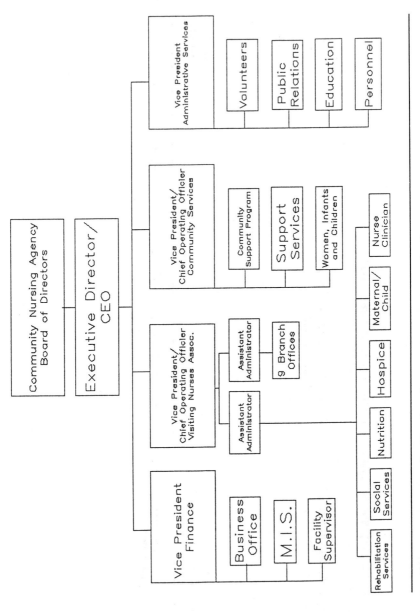

Exhibit 11-1 Community Nursing Agency corporate organization.

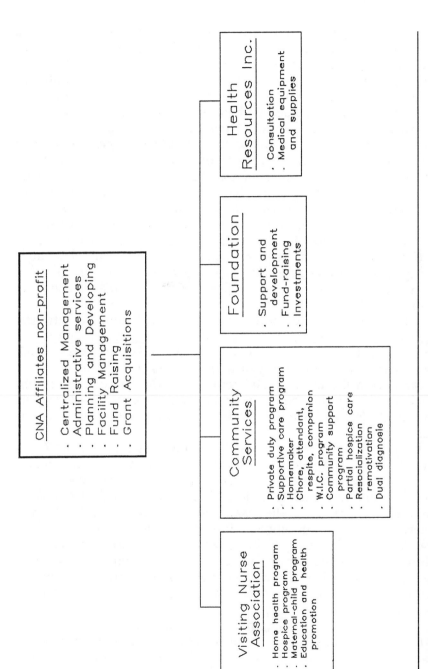

Exhibit 11-2 Community Nursing Agency corporate functions.

example, the advisory board of one of the branch offices held a meeting with the CEO to protest the pooling of United Way grants from the separate counties. The manager of that office did nothing to support the CEO's position at the meeting. Thus, her loyalty was interpreted by the CEO to be with the local board, not the agency.

The culture of the agency had long been dominated by professional pride. A strong sense of the autonomous role of the community nurse as a client advocate and case manager was a clear factor in the mode of nursing practice employed and the management structure. The visiting nurses, all R.N.s, were viewed as primary nurses or case managers in that they assumed responsibility for coordinating and monitoring the implementation of patient care plans. In addition to providing nursing services directly, the nurses arranged for physical and occupational therapy visits, made contacts with attending physicians, supervised nurses' aides, counseled family caregivers, and completed the documentation required for reimbursement of services. The nursing care plan format is shown in Exhibit 11-3.

The primary nurse concept requires considerable decentralization of control for the management of nursing care. Traditional management of community nursing has involved centralized scheduling whereby a daily itinerary or quota of "tickets" for client visits is picked up in the morning and returned at the end of each day by each nurse. In this now outdated, alternative style, supervisors managed cases and nurses provided a more limited range of nursing care services.

There seemed to be no doubt in anyone's mind at the Community Nursing Agency that the primary, community nurse model was the state of the art. This decentralized model was preferable for both patient care quality and staff satisfaction. Staff felt patients were well supervised in their own homes and the nurses' status was elevated above the traditional view of the nurse as the physician's handmaiden. Though job stress was greater with the increased responsibility of the primary nurse role, turnover among the agency's nurses was quite low. Community, home-based care focused on the whole patient in his or her environment and was considered to be nursing at its best.

The community nursing philosophy was evident in many ways. All of the executives except the financial officer were nurses and were long-term employees who had risen through the ranks. The nursing assessment form used by the agency (Exhibit 11-4) reflected a nursing diagnosis format with physician orders included as only

COMMUNITY NURSING AGENCY CARE PLAN

Client: _____
Primary: _____
Admission Nurse: _____

Agency Number: _____
Physician: _____
Physician Phone No.: _____

Status Code

R = resolved
O = ongoing

Date	Code	Health Problem	Diagnosis Etiology	Status	Objective Target Date	Interventions

Exhibit 11-3 Community Nursing Agency care plan.

COMMUNITY NURSING AGENCY NURSING ASSESSMENT
(not including codes)

Client:_____   Agency Number:_____

Environmental Domain   Observations/Description

    01   Neighborhood: Deficit
    02   Residence: Deficit
    03   Community Resource Utilization: Deficit

Physiological Domain

    04   Integument: Impairment
    05   Stimulation: Impairment
    06   Oxygenation: Impairment
    07   Circulation: Impairment
    08   Body temperature: Impairment
    09   Fluid and electrolyte:
    10   Nutrition: Impairment
    11   Bowel elimination: Impairment
    12   Urinary elimination: Impairment
    13   Sexuality: Alteration
    14   Mobility: Impairment
    15   Sleep/rest: Impairment
    16   Comfort: Alteration
    17   Self-care: Deficit

Interdependence Domain

    18   Communication: Impairment
    19   Interactional ability: Impairment
    20   Role: Alteration
    21   Self-concept: Alteration
    22   Thought: Alteration
    23   Mood expression: Impairment
    24   Coping ability: Impairment
    25   Learning: Dysfunction

Health Behaviors Domain

    26   Complications:
    27   Medical/technical Procedure:
    28   Health promotion: Deficit

Exhibit 11-4 Community Nursing Agency nursing assessment (not including codes).

one source of input. The visiting nurse was expected to exercise independent nursing judgement beyond following the physician's orders, i.e., initiating services required to relieve the patient's symptoms. In describing her historical vision for the agency's development, the chief executive officer stated, "I have always viewed skilled nursing as our central service and the other services—social work; physical, speech, and respiratory therapy; and nutritional counseling—as ancillary." Whereas hospitals, at least until recently, have been the "physician's workshop," the Community Nursing

Agency makes it very clear that, at its core, it is based on professional nursing practice.

Just as hospitals found that the prospective payment system required changes in physician behavior, the professional practice of nursing faced new constraints when managing home care in a cost-containment environment. Both home care nurses' and physicians' clinical judgements regarding the use of Medicare-reimbursed services required attention to strictures imposed by the cost-containment efforts of the Health Care Financing Administration (HCFA). Changes in hospital based physician care resulted from the implementation of the Tax Equity and Fiscal Responsibility Act of 1982 (TEFRA). The constraints faced by the home care industry were the result of regulatory changes gradually imposed between 1985 and 1987. Increasingly nurses' judgements about patient needs for services were being rejected by the Medicare intermediary. As the Chief Operating Officer of the Visiting Nurses' Association put it, "It's what I've always been proudest of—the primary nurse model. And now it's killing us."

Environmental Factors

Except for state Medicaid programs, the major environmental factors that have affected the growth of the home care industry were identified in the analysis by Van Gelder and Bernstein (1986). These factors include the following:

1. Medicare's home health and hospice benefits
2. Experimental payment systems
3. Growth of community-based models of care and technologies
4. State certificate-of-need policies
5. Growth in the over age 75 population
6. Private long-term care insurance
7. Medicare hospital prospective payment system.

In Pennsylvania, growth in the home care industry has been fueled primarily by the market opportunity provided by Medicare reimbursement and by the absence of certificate-of-need requirements. Pennsylvania reimburses for services provided to Medicaid clients on a flat rate basis, and rates remained frozen as they had been for several years.

Although only about 2 percent of Medicare expenditures are for home care, Medicare has been the major reimbursement source for home health benefits. The Omnibus Reconciliation Act of 1980 expanded the Medicare home care benefit as an alternative to more expensive inpatient care, made it easier for proprietary firms to enter the market and led to a major transformation of home care in Pennsylvania.

During the 1980s, the environment for established home health providers such as CNA changed in several significant ways. Their sole provider status was eroded by competitors including hospitals and health-related corporations with diverse interests and services which entered the home health field. As vertical integration became a major competitive strategy for many health care organizations in Pennsylvania, home health was seen as a wide open market. The capital investment needed to test a home health service was relatively small and no geographic market seemed too obscure. By the mid-1980s, the CNA had competitors encroaching on its market, one of which had entered into an exclusive referral arrangement with an area hospital. This arrangement was costly to CNA in terms of lost referrals. Referrals from physicians and hospitals are the fiscal life line of home health care agencies.

Secondly, federal initiatives to contain hospital costs had spillover effects for home care providers. Agency nurses were being asked to provide care beyond their technical capacity. "Sicker and quicker" hospital discharges meant an increased demand for skilled nursing and other services to assist patient transitions to self-care. Coincidentally, the HCFA began a series of regulatory measures designed to limit the use of the Medicare home care benefit to short-term, relatively acute care. While the number of clients needing home care remained stable or increased, the number of Medicare-reimbursed home visits was being reduced dramatically. The provision of profitable, supportive, non-nursing services also was curtailed. Even the most carefully managed agencies, which had balanced Medicare-reimbursed services (reimbursed at cost) with Medicaid-provided services (reimbursed at less than one-half of the actual cost), found themselves fiscally squeezed. Many new and some established home care providers went out of business.

Key Actors: The Administrative Team

Leading the "A-team," as the executive group referred to itself, was Ann Beardon, R.N., M.S.N., Chief Executive Officer (CEO), Community Nursing Agency Affiliates. Perceived by her subordinates as a highly articulate and intelligent woman, Beardon admitted that she is a perfectionist and could be difficult to work with at times. She had achieved positions of prominence in the community and in state and national professional organizations. Hired as director of the agency 15 years ago, she led its expansion into multiple sites, programs, new funding sources, and service arenas. The nursing staff spoke of her with remote admiration and a sense of trust in the well-being of the agency under her leadership. Managers at all levels were keenly aware of her power, appreciative of its authoritative base, and occasionally stunned by its autocratic side effects. In describing how Beardon had aided her transition from nursing to a management position, one administrator recalled the CEO's statement: "You can't make a mistake so big that I can't get you out of it." She knew every aspect of the business that she needed to know.

Catherine Downey, R.N., Chief Operating Officer (COO) of the Visiting Nurses Association had directed the VNA for four years before the reorganization which established her current position. Catherine began 13 years earlier with the agency as a visiting nurse. Staff nurses and supervisors related to her as one of them. She also was viewed as a tragic heroine, having sustained her career through a terminal illness in her immediate family. Downey felt considerable role confusion in her position as COO of the Visiting Nurses Association. While it was clear to her that there were aspects of her job that Beardon had not yet relinquished, Downey was unsure about how to establish her authority. She took management courses on her own time and believed that she had made some progress in diminishing her role as the "bottleneck" in the agency hierarchy. Downey frequently expressed the stress she experienced as her commitment to professional and high quality community nursing conflicted with the need to take the "bottom-line" view of the administrator.

Evelyn Frongello, R.N., Chief Operating Officer (COO), Community Services Program, was known to her colleagues as a "doer, not a dreamer." Frongello was appreciated by her peers and subordinates for her ability to implement ideas. While not trained in business or management, Frongello developed and implemented her programs like a true entrepreneur, occasionally too aggressively for some internal competitors.

Grace Harper, R.N., Vice President for Administrative Services, CNA Affiliates, acted as the chief of operations for the entire corporation. This spring and summer, Harper was heavily involved in a major building renovation and in orienting a new personnel director to the realties of managing in the nonprofit sector.

Ivan Jameson, C.P.A., Vice President for Finance, CNA Affiliates, was the only male administrator. He had grown accustomed to redoing his handwritten budgets on short notice and fixing furnaces in emergency situations.

The Problem of Increased Claim Denials

Home health care services provided to Medicare-eligible patients by certified providers are reimbursable on a per-visit fee basis. Skilled nursing, home health aide care, and other therapies are provided under Medicare if skilled nursing care is ordered by a physician and meets the criteria for medical necessity set forth by the HCFA. These criteria became more stringent as the prospective payment system took effect in reimbursing hospitals for acute care. The apparent fear that growth in home health care would offset savings derived from limiting the growth of inpatient care had led to a series of regulatory changes enacted through HCFA's fiscal intermediary organizations.

The changes resulted in increased numbers of claims for reimbursement for visits being denied on both technical and medical grounds. The agency's denial rate or the percentage of visits submitted to the HCFA intermediary and not reimbursed, had become a key financial indicator, as it had industry-wide. Prior to this summer, the agency had been operating under a waiver system which allowed providers whose denial rates remained under 2.5 percent to receive bimonthly estimated payments, thereby stabilizing cash flow.

At the June 15 meeting of the A-team, the administrative assistant in charge of third party reimbursement mechanisms presented a report. Her findings, though not entirely unexpected, elicited a somewhat startled response. Her report indicated that the denial rate had steadily risen from 1.5 percent last year to over 4.0 percent for the first quarter of this year. As a consequence, the agency would be taken "off waivers." These preset forward payments had continued several months after the denial rate had increased above the 2.5 percent standard, due to the time lag involved in appealing denials. The result was an overpayment of more than $80,000 which CNA would have to begin repaying immediately.

Other information provided included a review by the assistant administrator in charge of quality assurance of measures initiated to halt the problem of increasing numbers of visits being denied reimbursement. These measures included training sessions for nurses on documentation techniques to reduce the number of claim denials, memos to the branch office managers whenever policy changes from the intermediary were announced, and repeated and unsuccessful attempts to establish meaningful liaison with the Medicare inter- mediary reviewers (in Philadelphia) by telephone. There was some discussion of the possible reasons for the increased number of visits denied. The administrative assistant in charge of third party reim- bursement attributed much of the problem to nurses not using information provided at training sessions on preventing denials. For example, if a nurse failed to call a patient prior to making a visit and arrived at their home only to find a homebound patient absent, that and prior visits would likely be denied by the HCFA if the form was submitted for the current visit. There were numerous possible documentation inconsistencies that caused denials which in the past had been either overlooked or sought to be clarified by the inter- mediary.

Several team members commented that the primary nurse model might have to be reconsidered and that the agency might have to return to a more controlled medical model of care. The question was raised, "Can nursing assessment focus on financial as well as clinical data, or is that asking too much?" After a discussion of the moral implications of asking nurses to terminate cases earlier, Downey confessed she was getting really frustrated by the discussion. When Beardon asked, "What can we do to help you with this?" she had no suggestions. At the end of the meeting, Beardon appointed a task force to design a plan of action to stop the trend toward increasing denial rates. The task force included Downey, the quality assurance manager, the third-party liaison, and Downey's assistant administrator, who directly supervised the branch office managers.

Attempts to Decrease the Claim Denial Rate

Several weeks after the task force was appointed, an update on the denial problem was scheduled on the A-team meeting agenda. The other major agenda item involved setting budget priorities for the next fiscal year. Downey reported that she had visited the branch offices, met with the nursing staff, and attempted to explain the seriousness of the problem. She perceived that the nurses and the Branch office managers were stressed by the situation. Suddenly, the quality of services they had been encouraged to provide was considered inappropriate. Criticism of their record keeping performance added to their anger and frustration. Some of the branch office managers started special review processes to detect documentation errors though no one knew what the overall effect would be. This response to the problem was characterized as plugging leaks in a dam. New reasons for denying claims were produced by the intermediary as soon as staff were able to adjust and gain control over earlier errors. For example, with considerable effort, staff nurses were trained to comply with a revised interpretation of the "homebound" criteria for continued care. While this reeducation was underway, a new set of changes was being introduced as a basis upon which visits were denied. It appeared that this incremental and sporadic approach to problem-solving alone would not allow the agency to gain control over the denial problem.

Another strategy which the administrators expected would impact the denial rate was the implementation of computerized HCFA forms. Using these precoded forms for admission and recertification would drastically reduce the amount of narrative documentation completed by nurses, thereby reducing both the likelihood of technical errors and the discretion given to individual nurses in describing the processes of patient care. This strategy, like others, however, could not be evaluated for several months and neither could the effectiveness of the appeals process which took months or years to pursue in individual cases.

The Financial Crisis Worsens

In the weeks before the July 29 meeting, other facts had surfaced to complicate the situation. The number of visits being made by the VNA nurses had fallen below expected levels (Table 11-2). Twenty-six percent fewer Medicare visits were made in the first six months of the current year than were budgeted and 12 percent less than had been made in the first half of last year. This decrease was due to the reduction in the number of Medicare-reimbursable visits allowed per case as well as some encroachment of competitors on referral sources. Given that 75-80 percent of the agency's home

Table 11-2 Year-to-Date (YTD) visits by discipline, Visiting Nurse Association (June).

Discipline	Actual YTD	Budget YTD	Last year YTD
Nursing therapy	34,149	41,507	35,667
Physical therapy	2,425	5,148	4,269
Speech therapy	626	1,468	1,069
Occupational therapy	878	1,333	702
Medical social service	846	1,390	822
Home health aide	20,926	25,946	23,063
Maternal child	709	1,613	1,260
Hospice	2,138	2,373	1,920
Other	3	189	156
Total paid visits	62,700	80,968	68,938
Non-paid visits	3,037	3,946	4,045
Total visits-VNA	65,737	84,914	72,983
Medicare visits	46,411	62,787	53,146

visits were reimbursed by Medicare, this was perceived as being even more troublesome than the cash flow problem identified earlier. As the next year's budget projections took form, it became clear that reasonable productivity ratios (the number of visits per nurse per day) could not be achieved with current nurse staffing levels. Beardon was concerned, however, that eliminating nursing positions to reduce costs would be short-sighted given the much publicized, impending nursing shortage.

Review of monthly financial statements at the July 29 meeting showed that Medicaid-reimbursed visits had risen. Medicaid visits for nursing services were reimbursed by Pennsylvania at less than 50 percent of their cost. To control these losses, each branch office was assigned a monthly allotment in this year's budget from community donations to cover these contractual allowances. Several branch offices had exceeded their annual allotments by mid-year. Nurses were obviously charging visits to Medicaid which they knew would be denied by Medicare for those financially eligible. While in theory this is how Medicaid should be used, the provision of Medicaid services is as costly to home health agencies as it is to other providers in states where reimbursement levels are low. Thus, the failure of the agency to control the use of Medicaid was another factor deepening the agency's financial cash flow crisis. "The message we need to get out to the nurses," stated Beardon, "is that we are not going to endanger patients, but unless we are more selective in the number of Medicaid visits we make, we may not be around to serve anyone." Ivan Jameson, the agency's financial director for the past decade, announced he had accepted a position elsewhere. While his stated reason for leaving was pursuit of new opportunities, Beardon felt the complexity of financial management under the new corporate structure exceeded his capacities. Jameson gave the agency a month's notice. It was clear that even a financial wizard could not resolve this crisis quickly.

On July 21, the branch office managers held a meeting discussing concerns about their place in the organization. The meeting was held at the suggestion of Downey who felt these managers needed to "ventilate." Although they embraced their newly articulated marketing role, they did not feel they could perform this function while providing the increased clinical supervision demanded. Clinical supervision included review of 10 percent of all case records for quality assurance and utilization review and to monitor the appropriateness of service. In recent months, additional chart reviews of diagnoses flagged as most likely to result in denials had been added to the list of branch office manager duties. Though each manager was a nurse without managerial training, their clear preference was to move out of the clinical supervisor role and more substantively into management. They requested that offices with higher volume be assigned clinical supervisors. A-team members were frustrated by the request, seeing the negative impact of such non reimbursable staff functions on the agency's efficiency. In short, it was not the supportive, creative, and loyal response to the financial crisis which they hoped would emerge.

The Team Develops Financial Strategies

At the August 5 meeting of the A-team, the agenda contained a single item—identify options for easing the agency's impending cash flow crisis. The issue went well beyond the balance sheets, however, as next year's budget unfolded. Beardon began the meeting by stating the importance of keeping the perspective that the agency was still, as it had always been, financially healthy. "The current situation," she reiterated, "is extremely serious, but we are not in danger of going under and I want the staff to know that. Any rumors to the contrary will only help our competitors." Having set that tone, Beardon left the meeting to take a phone call from the director of the state association of home care agencies. This association was preparing a major organized protest to the legislature regarding Medicaid reimbursement and Beardon had definite ideas she wanted to have represented.

During her 20-minute absence, the group became impatient. The administrators responded unenthusiastically when Grace Harper attempted to focus on the agenda. The consensus was that it would be a waste of effort to proceed without Beardon. When Beardon returned, it was clear to her that no progress had been made, so she went to the newsprint stand and initiated a group discussion, asking each person around the table how she/he would reduce costs and increase revenues.

The options suggested by team members for reducing costs included the following:

1. Beardon: eliminate all staff nurse positions and substitute an all PRN (as needed) nursing staff
2. Downey: reduce the number of nurse positions

3. Frongello: close one or two of the smaller offices

4. Harper: reduce the number of non-nurse positions

5. Jameson: stop serving Medicaid patients for the remainder of the year

6. Harper: eliminate a vice-president position

The suggestions on how to increase revenues were more upbeat.

1. Beardon: use in-house nurse reviewers to restore the Medicare denial rate to 1.5 percent or less

2. Harper: increase referrals by having branch office managers intensify physician liaison functions

3. Frongello: market to increase the amount of private duty nursing and other fee-for-service programs offered

4. Jameson: increase rates for services

5. Beardon: launch a major fund-raising drive

The activity budget projections for next year were presented by Jameson. Based on this year's performance, the total number of agency visits for next year was projected at 121,000 (some 40,000 less than this year's budget), with the bulk of the loss occurring in the Medicare-reimbursed VNA visits. After some discussion, it was agreed that this conservative estimate would be necessary as a basis for planning. This meant that adjustments in programs would be required for the remainder of this year, and next year's budget requests from the programs and branch offices would have to reflect downsizing.

At the conclusion of the August 5 meeting, Beardon directed the A-team members to come to the meeting next week with their recommendations for staff and/or program reductions and new initiatives to increase revenues in their programs. While the VNA was the loser in this current situation, the problem was clearly one shared by each of the executives.

After the meeting, Beardon pondered her own next steps. She was aware of the strain the executives were under. They had experience managing growth, not shrinkage, and the idea of laying off staff was profoundly unsettling. As always, the dilemma of how far to push her own agenda was there. The A-team members needed to develop confidence in themselves as executives, yet they seemed unwilling to risk her disapproval. The nursing staff needed to be convinced that agency survival was as critical an objective as quality of care. Their documentation precision and certain professional judgement patterns had to change. Who could most effectively provide this leadership while at the same time managing downsizing?

Part V

Strategic Planning and Community Relations

Introduction

Donna Lind Infeld

Strategic planning includes evaluation of internal and external resources and opportunities and collection of appropriate data to decide on new directions for an organization. Marketing new ventures is closely related to the strategic planning process. Some cases in this section focus on strategic decisions to expand long-term care services within an existing organization. Others focus on strategic redirection of existing services in light of changing environmental conditions.

"Strategic Planning in a Continuing Care Retirement Community" examines the recommendations of a consultant hired to develop a strategic plan. A church-sponsored retirement community must decide whether to broaden its range of long-term care services. Personalities, governing board relations, and financial concerns influence this case.

"Conflicting Strategies for Market Expansion: Hospital-Based Home Health Services" examines strategic planning at a hospital which must decide whether to develop a home health care program. In a competitive market for home health care, the hospital is confronted with issues of certificate of need, financial viability, and alternative investment options.

Sunny Acres Villa, Inc. is placed on a "Contractual Tightrope" due to the difficulties of operating a facility with life care contracts.

Marketing is an important aspect of the strategic efforts facing this facility.

Other cases in the book can also be examined for their strategic planning potential. For example, most of the organizations described have developed a firm foundation for strategic planning; that is, they have a defined philosophy of care, mission statement, or other principle governing operations. Those facilities that do not, clearly need to develop such statements. In the current competitive health care environment, strategic planning capabilities may determine the survival of many long-term care programs and services.

Case 12

Strategic Planning in a Continuing Care Retirement Community[*]

William E. Aaronson

William E. Aaronson, Ph.D., is Assistant Professor, Department of Health and Medical Services Administration, Widener University.

Case Overview

Steve Cantwell was preparing for the next meeting of the Long Range Planning Committee of the board of directors of the Mueller-O'Keefe Memorial Home and Retirement Village. Steve was a consultant with a major independent long-term care consulting firm. He had been given the task of directing this project. It had been a difficult task from the beginning. Although he had dealt with similar situations in the past, this project presented some unique challenges.

The consulting firm for whom Steve worked dealt almost exclusively with not-for-profit long term care providers. The majority of clients were church sponsored or affiliated. Although well intentioned, governing board members of these types of providers were not always well informed about the current challenges and opportunities within the long-term care environment.

The Mueller-O'Keefe Home was one such church-related client. The home was affiliated with the Evangelical Free Church. All members of the board of directors, except one, were church

---

[*] Fictitious names of both the organization and individuals are used to ensure anonymity.

members. The church district executive was an *ex officio* board member. Although the board consisted of church members, the home was not sponsored by the church. The board was self-perpetuating and independent, but chose to maintain close ties with the church.

During a retreat, the board of directors had determined that they would require outside consulting services. They recognized their personal limitations when it came to the development, selection and implementation of alternative courses of action. Through a subcommittee, the Long Range Planning Committee, the consulting firm for whom Steve worked was retained. The consulting firm was to assist the home in developing a long range plan which included identification of new services and a capital development plan.

Steve felt comfortable working with this Board. All members whom he had met were dedicated to and concerned about the home. A few of the members were actually looking forward to entering the retirement village when the time would come to decide on their own postretirement moves.

Steve was approaching this latest meeting with a great deal of concern. The purpose of the meeting was to serve as a working session in which his report would be discussed and the feasibility of the action recommendations would be considered. He had spent considerable time researching the market, analyzing the organization, and developing alternatives that he felt fit both the Home's mission and the organization's abilities. His report was well prepared and appeared to be congruent with the board's perception of the home's mission. However, despite endless interviews with board members, staff, residents, competitors, and community representatives, and after extensive research on the alternatives, he wondered whether the board would approve and respond to his recommendations. He knew that *he* had every reason to be confident in his counsel, or did he?

The History and Development of the Home

The Mueller-O'Keefe Memorial Home was founded in 1905 when Dr. Robert Mueller bequeathed a large brick farmhouse and 90 acres of ground to a benevolent organization of members of the Evangelical Free Church. The purpose of the bequest was to establish a home for aged church members. The Evangelical Free Church "Old Folks Home," as it was called, became well established in the local community. The home is located in a rural setting near a small city in Ohio. Two wings were added to the original farmhouse in the 1930s, due to an increasing number of requests for admission.

The home continued to care exclusively for members of the Evangelical Free Church until 1951. Due to the fine reputation of the home and in response to some financial difficulties, Mr. Patrick O'Keefe, a prominent local industrialist, established a 25-year endowment. Mr. O'Keefe was Roman Catholic. The purpose of the endowment was to ensure financial stability, to allow expansion of facilities, and to encourage the home to open admissions to non-Free Church members. The endowment principal became fully available to the home last year.

The 1950s brought additional changes. The board began to recognize that residents of the home were requiring more nursing care. The home never had an empty bed. When a resident died, the bed was quickly filled. However, when residents moved into the home they were generally in poorer health than in the past. Plans were initiated to build a nursing care wing onto the Old Folks Home. A 100-bed addition was built in the early 1960s which brought the total complement to 140 beds.

Another major innovation for the Mueller-O'Keefe Home occurred in the 1960s. The first retirement cottage was built in 1962, initially as a house for the administrator, whose presence at the home was increasingly required. He retired soon after the house was built, and he was allowed to remain there. When it became known that the grounds could be used for retirement living, retired couples began to apply for lots where they could build houses to their liking. The retirement "cottages" (single-family ranch style houses) would become property of the home upon completion. The original residents were offered life care contracts in return for the donation of the constructed cottage to the home. This experiment with life care contracts was short lived, due to an early recognition of the future potential for financial liability.

One current resident of the nursing home is the last such person to have held a life care contract. She is 96 and the cost of her care long ago exceeded the value of her property. However, the home continues to honor her contract by providing free care. In the mid-1960s the first "continuing care" contract was written. Contingent liability for care was to be limited to the construction cost or resale value of the cottages. Residents would be given preference for admission to nursing care.

A row of eight apartments was added in the early 1970s. These apartments are similar in appearance to single-story townhouses. In the late 1970s, the first attempt to plan within the retirement village took place. An architect was hired to design a state-of-the-art quadriplex, similar to cottage construction taking place at other retirement communities. However, when the building was completed, it did not fit with the predominant design of the community—it resembled an Aspen ski lodge. The home had difficulty selling the cottages. This reinforced the board's belief that "seat of the pants" decisions generally resulted in better outcomes, a belief that many of the Board members continued to hold. However, haphazard land development had created its own problems, primarily involving efficient land use and seweage disposal.

In the 1970s the ratio of nursing care to residential care in the Old Folks Home increased rapidly. In 1970 only 53 beds were certified for nursing care. By 1977 all of the beds (100) in the nursing care building were certified. In 1985, two additional beds were added bringing the total nursing care beds to 102. These new beds were to be held in reserve for the use of the retirement village residents. Personal care beds remained fixed at 40. They have continued to be located in the Mueller farmhouse. The buildings were modest, especially when compared to competing long-term care facilities.

By the 1980s the home's staff began to recognize that many of the home's residents had developed Alzheimer's disease or related dementias. Individuals in early and middle stages of the disease were particularly difficult to manage in a congregate living arrangement due to behavioral manifestations which the staff observed to be annoying to other residents. Therefore, a separate unit for confused, ambulatory residents was initiated. The Alzheimer's disease unit quickly developed a reputation for providing exceptional care. The Administrator, Mr. Clark, reported that the board was particularly interested in expanding this unit. However, he personally was uncertain about this option. Although it would certainly bring publicity and possibly additional sources of funding, it might also result in the home developing an image as a mental health facility, which might have negative consequences on future admissions.

According to Mr. Clark, the home had maintained a reputation for excellent basic care throughout its history. The Evangelical Free Church is a service-oriented denomination which draws its social philosophy from New Testament teachings. Church members are traditionally conscientious objectors and, like the Quakers and the Amish, are excused from military service when a national draft is in effect. Outward expressions of Christian values among administration, staff, and residents were very evident to Steve. According to

Mr. Clark, this atmosphere, rather than the physical environment and other amenities, had been the key factor attracting residents to the home.

According to the board chairman, Mr. Polk, two important consequences had resulted. Many current residents of the retirement village and nursing care had parents, grandparents, aunts, uncles, and siblings who are or have been residents of the home. Every resident of the home had heard of it by word of mouth and usually were intimately aware of it when making their post-retirement move decisions. Secondly, the home has been frequently remembered in the wills of residents or relatives of residents who were pleased with the care received.

By the end of last May, the home's investment assets, held in the form of securities, were valued at approximately $3.5 million. Another $230,000 was held in a low interest savings account. Net fixed assets were valued at $1.7 million for a fund balance of $5.6 million. The home did not have any long-term or short-term debt. This very positive financial picture, combined with an ever-growing demand for the services of the home, convinced the board of directors that some future-oriented growth strategies were required. The Long Range Planning Committee was charged with the responsibility for developing alternative uses of the available funds.

Mr. O'Donnell, Long Range Planning Committee Chairman, stated that the committee immediately ran into problems. First, the board was not solidly behind any planning efforts. The home's growth in the past had been essentially unplanned. "Seat of the pants" decision making appeared to have worked well. Few freestanding nursing homes or retirement centers were as financially healthy as the home. Also, the debacle of the "ski lodge" cottages was seen as the result of the only planning endeavor ever undertaken.

Secondly, many board members were opposed to incurring long-term debt for any reason. Mr. Polk, who in the 1930s had seen what over-extension of credit could do to a business, was especially opposed. It soon became apparent that without debt, the home's options were severely limited.

Thirdly, the home did not have a formally adopted mission statement. There was disagreement within the board as to whether one was necessary, since they had managed for 80 years without one. However, it did not seem likely that the board would agree on any plans since they were divided on issues related to the basic mission (who was to be served and how) and church relations. As a church-affiliated home, a common mission was recognized as important by the board chairman and by some members of the committee who were trying to focus on acceptable growth options.

The Consultants Begin Their Analyses

In the midst of these impending changes and conflicting opinions, the consulting firm was hired. The first meeting that Steve had with the Long Range Planning Committee revealed several things. The initial proposal he submitted would have to be modified in response to some committee members' concerns. The chairman of the board, Mr. Polk, had objected to some of the terminology in particular. They would prefer to be called a home, not a facility. The committee requested that statistics and charts be kept to a minimum. They preferred to be given recommendations in common language. Finally, Steve had noted with some concern that the administrator, Tom Clark, was exceptionally quiet throughout the meeting. Despite the key role he would need to play in the planning process and in the implementation of any plans, his interactions and responses were subdued.

Steve was given a free hand by the committee to develop the long-range plan. The consulting contract stated that this plan would be developed through a process which ended with the presentation to the committee of several alternative strategies. Useful decision criteria were also to be developed. However, it was made clear to the board and the committee that they were to make the final strategic choice. The consultants were to provide the professional expertise in areas of market analysis and internal organizational review. That knowledge, in conjunction with an in-depth analysis of the organization, was to result in the proposal of strategic alternatives that would be feasible and consistent with the organization's abilities.

Steve observed that the Long Range Planning Committee was determined to take a passive role in the process. Mr. Polk, although not a member of the committee, took the most active role. Mr. Clark confided to Steve that, although Mr. Polk appeared to dominate the board and the committee, he was actually very democratic. He believed that if other members would exert themselves, Mr. Polk would yield to the will of the majority. Mr. Clark stated that he could see no reason why Mr. Polk's philosophy would be any different under these circumstances.

Mr. Polk had some very definite ideas about what should or should not be done. He viewed the rather substantial endowment and the excellent financial position of the home to be the result of his prudent financial management. Mr. Polk also served as the treasurer which can be equated with the position of chief financial officer for the home. In addition, he was the vice president for finance of a family owned furniture business. His financial acumen was developed through a 45-year career with the furniture company. Experience taught him to be wary of debt of any kind.

In reviewing four years worth of balance sheets (Table 12-1), Steve noted that the accounts payable balance was identical ($10,360) at the close of each period. When questioned, Mr. Polk said that it was a fictitious amount. All bills had been paid upon receipt. Consequently, the actual balance on the books in accounts payable at the end of the accounting period was zero. However, the state Medicaid program auditors reportedly would not accept a zero balance.

Steve had initiated the planning process knowing that implementation of any plan would be problematic. Any program development, no matter how modest, would result in debt being incurred. Further, due to lack of depth in administration, organizational and management development would be required regardless of which direction was taken. The process was initiated with an organizational review, an analysis of current residents, a demographic analysis, and a financial review. A competitor analysis was also conducted which included tours of and interviews at competing retirement communities and nursing homes. Staff from the area agency on aging and the health systems agency were interviewed as well. Finally, residents, staff, and board members were selected for more extensive interviews.

Based on the findings from the first part of the study, sessions were to be conducted with the Long Range Planning Committee in which the working papers would be discussed and which would serve as the basis for preparation of the final document. The results of the working documents are summarized in the following sections.

Organizational Review

The board of directors has final responsibility for the operations of the home. The daily operational responsibilities for all facilities and programs are delegated to the administrator, Mr. Clark. Responsibility for the financial management of the home remained

Table 12-1 Comparative balance sheets.

	This year	Last year	2 years ago	3 years ago
Assets				
Current				
cash	$ 231,149	$ 192,013	$ 127,747	$ 77,899
Acct. rec.	159,223	157,975	145,189	190,092
Inventory	400	400	400	400
Prepaid ins.	29,015	10,921	13,632	5,511
Total	419,787	361,309	286,963	273,902
Non-current				
Agent acct.	1,557,386	1,307,386	748,473	642,707
Trust acct.	1,901,122	1,651,122	1,388,735	1,193,165
Total	$3,458,508	$2,958,508	$2,137,208	$1,835,872
Fixed Assets				
Land	$ 10,284	$ 10,284	$ 10,284	$ 10,284
Buildings	1,702,214	1,699,214	1,671,621	1,666,787
Water/sewer	204,747	204,747	204,747	178,885
Vehicles	105,532	104,846	54,356	54,356
Equipment	437,171	422,663	386,970	363,487
Cottages	303,452	254,050	230,224	150,494
Total	2,763,400	2,695,804	2,558,202	2,424,293
Deprec.	1,073,784	1,052,207	998,329	953,807
Net Fixed Assets	$1,689,616	$1,643,597	$1,559,873	$1,470,486
Total Assets	$5,567,911	$4,963,414	$3,984,044	$3,580,260

Liabilities & Fund Balance				
Acct. pay.	10,360	10,360	10,360	$ 10,360
Payroll	39,410	47,037	33,384	29,513
Tax pay.	5,368	5,171	4,912	4,441
Total	55,147	62,577	48,665	44,323
Reserves				
Res. care	(57,505)	(54,137)	(47,388)	(41,451)
Memorials	30,239	30,105	27,920	26,819
Res. exp.	(6,679)	1,372	(703)	0
Total	(33,945)	(22,660)	(20,177)	(14,632)
Fund Balance	5,546,709	4,923,497	3,955,556	3,550,569
Total Liab. & Fund Balance	$5,567,911	$4,963,414	$3,984,044	$3,580,260

with the board chairman, Mr. Polk. The financial analyst and the bookkeeper, although reporting to Mr. Clark on paper, actually reported directly to Mr. Polk. Mr. Clark did have mid-level managers who were responsible for operations within the nursing unit. However, he took full responsibility for the retirement village.

According to Mr. Polk, the board allowed Mr. Clark considerable latitude in running the home. The previous board chairman (Mr. Polk's predecessor) had allowed the previous administrator (Mr. Clark's predecessor) very little room for decision making. The home experienced some financial difficulties under the former chairman and administrator. Consequently, about ten years ago, that board chairman was asked to resign. The administrator was asked to resign as well later that year. Mr. Polk was then selected as the new chairman and hired Mr. Clark as the administrator. Mr. Polk and Mr. Clark had been in their current positions approximately ten years. They were both members of the same Evangelical Free Church congregation and had known each other for a considerably longer period of time. Substantial trust between the two men was apparent.

Steve observed that Mr. Clark exhibited little imagination in dealing with the home's operations. He also observed that Mr. Clark did an excellent job with the day-to-day management of the home. Employees were productive and contented with their work. Residents were generally well satisfied with their care. The home enjoyed an excellent reputation for the provision of high-quality basic care. Mr. Clark fostered the kind of work environment that made this possible. However, he did not appear to have a thorough understanding of the current long term-care environment, in particular, the concept of a continuum of care. Mr. Clark did not seem to recognize the need to bridge the gap between total independence and total dependence of retirement village residents. He stated that he could not understand why the retirement village residents were becoming more vociferous in their demands for services.

Steve observed that, financially, the home was generally well managed. Mr. Polk appeared to be a prudent and well intentioned individual who had managed to reverse the financial problems of the 1970s. This was done without the benefit of a high powered financial management staff. However, Mr. Polk also appeared to lack an understanding of the distinctions between financial management of a not-for-profit health care facility and that of a small, for-profit business. This was particularly apparent to Steve in the way that accounts were defined and segregated. The home actually had two equity accounts—capital contributions and retained earnings—which Steve combined into one account, the fund balance, for the purposes of the financial review. Fund accounting techniques were not evident. All accounts were integrated despite restrictions placed on certain funds. The distinct financial management needs of the continuing care facility were also not recognized by the home's financial manager. Planning for future financial stability was difficult as a consequence.

Resident Profile

The home provided services at three levels of care. Each level of care had a distinct resident profile.

The retirement village housed residents living in thirty-six units. Twenty-four of the units were single-family homes. The residents tended to be atypical of those residing in other continuing care retirement communities. The average resident age on admission was 70.6 years compared to a national average of 76 years. The average current age was 75.7 years compared to mature communities where the average age approximates 82 years (Table 12-2). Thus, the retirement village had a relatively young resident population. Close to one-half of the residents were members of the Evangelical Free Church (Table 12-3). Residents also tended to originate from distances further from the home than is typical (Table 12-4).

The nursing and personal care units were more typical of other church related nursing homes. The average age on admission (81 years) and the average current age (86 years) were comparable to national averages. Approximately 30 percent of nursing care and 25 percent of residential care residents were members of the Evangelical Free Church. This was similar to the experience of other denominational homes. However, more residents had entered from areas outside of the typical ten-mile radius from the home than would be expected of homes in areas of similar population density.

Despite the home's lack of promotional efforts, the nursing and residential care units and the retirement village remained full. Although 43 percent of the current residents' care was paid through the Medicaid program (Table 12-5), 90 percent had entered as self-pay residents. According to Mr. Clark, the high rate of conversion from self-pay to Medicaid was most likely due to the long lengths of stay in nursing care (4.5 years compared to a national average of just over two years). Mr. Clark further stated that Medicaid, as a percent of payer mix, would be higher if the home's

Table 12-2 Resident age characteristics (average age).

In-house Residents: December Last Year and National Data

Level of Care	Age at Admission (yrs.)	Age at Admission (national)	Current Age (yrs.)	National Average Age
Nursing Care*	81.0	N/A	86.0	N/A
Personal Care	82.0	N/A	86.0	N/A
Retirement Village**	70.0	76	75.7	82

*The age distribution of nursing home residents is skewed due to the ICF/MR program (facilities for the mentally retarded). According to the American College of Health Care Administrators Ready Reference Service, the current age is similar to the national experience, but the average length of stay at the Mueller-O'Keefe Home is approximately 3 years longer than the national average.

**82 years is the average age for retirement communities that opened between 1963 and 1973. *Source:* American Association of Homes for the Aging (1987). *Continuing Care Retirement Communities: An Industry in Action.*

Table 12-3 Religious preference by level of care.

Religious Preference	Nursing Care No.	Pct.	Personal Care No.	Pct.	Ret. Village No.	Pct.
	Level of Care					
Evangelical Free Church	29	29.0%	8	24.2%	16	47.2%
Methodist	27	27.0	13	39.4	5	14.7
Other Christian	40	40.0	12	36.4	8	23.4
None	4	4.0	0	0.0	5	14.7
Total	100	100.0%	33	100.0%	34	100.0%

Table 12-4 Resident origin by level of care–in-house residents: December 31, last year.

Prior Residence	Nursing Care No.	Pct.	Personal Care No.	Pct.	Ret. Village No.	Pct.
	Level of Care					
Home county	68	66.7%	26	76.5%	15	44.1%
Contiguous counties	20	19.6	6	17.7	3	8.8
Other	14	13.7	2	5.9	16	47.1
Total	102	100.0%	34	100.0%	34	100.0%

Table 12-5 Nursing care utilization profile by payer classification.

Year	Self-Pay		Medicaid	
	Pt. days	Pct.	Pt. Days	Pct.
Last year	21,731	59.5%	14,773	40.5%
2 years ago	20,407	57.7	15,383	42.3
3 years ago	22,102	60.6	14,368	39.4

private pay rates were equivalent to other nursing homes in the area. "Many of our residents are not well off. We want to give them the best care we can at the lowest rates so that we don't use up their assets any faster than necessary."

Financial Review

The home appeared to be on firm financial footing. Results of the financial statement analyses are presented in Table 12-6. Declining net revenues were noted two and three years ago. According to Mr. Polk, this trend resulted from the board's decisions not to raise rates during each of those years. However, a rate increase was put into effect at the end of last year which resulted in an increase in net revenue during the opening months of this year.

The home had adopted a rate policy for nursing care that was considered to be unique in the nursing home industry. Private rates were to be set no higher than Medicaid rates for the same patient services classification. This was directly related both to the basic care philosophy and to the social philosophy of the Evangelical Free Church. Mr. Clark stated that this policy actually resulted in the home having to refund money to the state's Medicaid program last year when the cost reports were analyzed and the state auditors realized that the rate setting commission had increased Medicaid rates to the home, but the private rates had not been increased by the board. Federal law does not permit Medicaid rates to exceed self pay rates.

Table 12-6 Comparative statement of revenues and expenses annualized.

	This year	Last year	2 years ago
Operating Revenues			
Resident care fees			
Personal care	$ 324,408	$ 312,927	$ 319,186
Self-pay ICF	1,094,658	1,020,978	978,382
Medicaid ICF	729,772	683,162	698,229
Other operating rev.	50,070	47,131	35,880
Total	$2,198,908	$2,064,198	$2,031,677
Operating Expenses			
Emp. compensation	$1,720,057	$1,702,209	$1,636,782
Supplies	112,010	107,723	108,080
Maintenance	78,940	69,510	64,694
Utilities	97,295	91,753	91,059
Prof. development	4,107	6,204	4,383
Prof. services	36,785	35,652	34,757
Insurance	37,099	35,074	17,608
Miscellaneous	4,282	4,625	3,174
Total	$2,090,575	$2,049,830	$1,960,537
Depreciation	73,470	62,704	44,522
Total Expenses	$2,164,045	$2,112,534	$2,005,059
Gain (loss) from operations	35,394	(48,335)	26,618
Non-operating rev.	131,400	72,619	72,705
Net income for period	$166,263	$ 24,283	$ 99,323

The retirement village residents, although not guaranteed care according to their contracts, were guaranteed a partial payment source for care based on their entrance fees. Entrance fees were to be depreciated over a 12-year period with the undepreciated balance available to pay for nursing care if the resident should permanently transfer to the nursing home. Steve became quite concerned when he could not track the entrance fees. Consequently, he could not accurately calculate the home's potential liabilities for care. The resident care reserve fund appeared to cover only residents who had actually transferred to nursing care. When questioned, Mr. Polk became defensive about this procedure. He stated that fees were deposited directly into one of the trust accounts. Resident care was provided according to the contracts and no problems had occurred to date.

The agent and trust accounts were administered by a local bank. There had been dramatic growth in these accounts in recent years. There were two sources for growth. First, donations had increased in recent years. However, the more important source of fund growth was related to the increase in value of the portfolio holdings. The holdings were re-valued to current market levels at the end of each period. Although the portfolio was diversified, the account balances were sensitive to changes in financial markets.

Environmental Analysis

There were two competing continuing care retirement communities in the home's primary service area. Mueller-O'Keefe's entrance and maintenance fees are lower than the others (Table 12-7). There were also nine nursing homes in competition for residents at that level of care (Table 12-8). The most significant finding was that the home's rates at all levels of care were the lowest in the county. Steve noted with some concern the differences in monthly maintenance

Table 12-7 Continuing Care retirement communities.

Community	Entrance Fees			Maintenance Fees (monthly)
Mueller-O'Keefe (church-related)	Cottages Apts.	– –	$55,000 25,000	$ 20
The Woods (church-related)	Cottages Apts.	– –	$70,500 47,500	$130
Luther Village (church-related)	Cottages	–	$60,000	$120

Table 12-8 Licensed nursing homes–primary service area.

Facility	Beds Nsg. care/Pers. care		Nursing Care Rates (per diem)
Mueller-O'Keefe (church-related)	102	40	Semi.–$46 Priv. –$47–$49
Andover Manor (for-profit)	221	0	Semi –$57–$59 Priv. –$59–$64
Clifton Home (for-profit)	49	0	Semi.–$50
County Home (government)	51	0	Semi.–$50–$60
The Court (for-profit)	160	0	Semi –$71–$74
Greywood Memorial (for-profit)	37	17	Semi.–$49
The Woods (church-related)	100	45	Semi.–$51 Priv. –$51
Luther Village (church-related)	88	0	Semi.–$58–$60 Priv. –$61
Methodist Home (church-related)	150	0	Semi.–$58–$65 Priv. –$68
Advent Hall (church-related)	97	0	Semi.–$53–$56 Priv. –$61
Total	1,053	102	

fees among the retirement communities. He had discussed this informally with Mr. Clark upon first reviewing the internal rate structure. Mr. Clark recognized that the fees were nowhere near adequate to cover costs. However, he stated that the board was more concerned about those living in the retirement village who could not afford the $120 per month that other communities charged. Mr. Clark felt that $120 was outrageous and that the other communities could not justify that amount. Steve also noted that the home's physical plant was more modest than the competitors' facilities.

The demographic analysis revealed several things that explained, to some extent, the competitive advantage of the home. First, there were few vacant beds in the county. Even those patients capable of self-pay for extended periods of time were having difficulty finding a nursing home bed. The home was located in an area characterized by a rapidly expanding elderly population. However, housing values and elderly income were below the state and national averages. Also, a higher percentage than expected of the oldest old lived alone—a situation that resulted in heavy demand for nursing home care. In the adjacent city, close to 50 percent of those older than age 75 lived alone, compared to approximately one-third on a national basis. The demographic and economic profiles also explained the slow growth that was experienced by the retirement village.

Interviews

Mr. Tom Clark, Administrator. "The retirement village residents are taking an increasing amount of my time. Without an assistant administrator, it is becoming more difficult to deal with problems caused by increasing age and decreasing independence. They pay a $20 per month maintenance fee. I can't provide all of the services that they expect on that amount.

"We emphasize excellent basic care in the nursing home. We intend to be the highest quality, lowest cost home in the county. Our philosophy of care is based on Christian principles. I don't want to deplete our residents' hard-earned savings. We figure that they will be on Medicaid soon enough, so why hurry the process. That is why we don't set self-pay rates above the Medicaid rate. We also aren't tempted to treat residents any differently based on payer status.

"Relations with the church have not always been smooth. The ladies' auxiliary, consisting largely of area church members, has made significant contributions both financially and in volunteer time. However, some pastors have been reluctant to become involved in the activities that we sponsor for the ladies' auxiliary, such as an annual barbecue and periodic breakfast meetings. We would like to have more involvement from the church.

"In the past, funds were severely limited. Construction was not always the highest quality. Maintenance costs are going up as a consequence. We may need to replace certain facilities in the future. The farmhouse may not be considered safe for residents at some point. However, due to the historical significance of the building, we would want to continue to utilize it."

Mrs. Hancock, Director of Nursing. "Care requirements are increasing across the board. We have had to increase our R.N. staff as a consequence. Of particular concern are the retirement village residents. A few of them should be in nursing care now. We end up providing free care on emergency bases when they can't get to their personal physicians.

"We don't know enough about their care requirements. This may be more of a problem in the future, especially if people are older when they first enter the retirement village or the personal care facility. We should be more aware of the medical care that they are receiving from their personal physicians. I don't have the time to make the contacts myself, even if the residents gave me permission to make contact."

Miss Webb, Director of Social Services. "People seeking admissions are generally older and sicker at each level of care. Nursing home beds are filled as soon as they are vacated. Most residents come from home or from other nursing homes. I seldom have a bed when the hospital social worker calls. She calls me anyway to see if I might have a bed, since the nursing home beds in this area are generally in short supply. The hospital has added its own skilled nursing care unit, but this isn't adequate to provide care for the many discharges who will require long-term care, rather that postacute extended care.

"People only leave the retirement village when they absolutely cannot care for themselves and, then, go directly to nursing care. We are supposed to have two beds in reserve for the retirement village. However, it doesn't always work out. Personal care would be better than remaining in independent living, but the residents don't care for the accommodations there."

Mr. Polk, Chairman, Board of Directors. "The local congregation of the Evangelical Free Church to which I belong has generously supported the home. Most board and ladies' auxiliary members also belong to my congregation. I'm not sure how much benefit increased church involvement would have, since other congregations have not been as financially generous.

"We're not sure how we should set our priorities. In particular, we would like to know how we can best use our available funds. However, I don't think it is appropriate to jeopardize our residents' security by incurring debt. I know of homes that have had financial difficulties due to overextending debt. If the board decides to finance growth through debt, I may need to reconsider my position on the board.

"I've suggested several mission statements, but the board has not decided which, if any, to adopt. Many feel that a mission statement might be too rigid. Obviously, our policies reflect the Christian mission of service on which this home was founded. We just don't have it written down."

Mr. O'Donnell, Chair, Long Range Planning Committee. "We need your help in planning for the future. We don't know enough about the different approaches to growth. We do know that if we grow, it has to be slow and planned. I don't like debt, but if we need it to meet our goals than we should do it. That's why we hired you. We also need to agree on our mission. We know that we want to serve the elderly and especially Evangelical Free Church elderly, but we also don't want to discriminate against those of other Christian denominations.

"Our buildings may need to be replaced in the future and we need to be prepared for that. Also, growth in the retirement village needs to be better planned."

Mrs. Ruth, Board Member. "We need to have closer ties to the Evangelical Free Church. It is not so much the financial support that they give, but the anchor that the church provides. That is, the church is where we go to assure that what we are doing is consistent with Christian social teaching and allows us to share our experience with others who have similar concerns."

Mrs. Jones, Nursing Home Ombudsman, Area Agency on Aging. "I hear only positive things. This is the only nursing home in my territory from which I have received no complaints since I was hired into this position two years ago."

Mr. and Mrs. Miller, Retirement Village Residents. "We love the single-family homes and the community spirit here. Nursing care is excellent. We know that if we really need care that the nursing home will provide good care. We are growing older and may need help with daily activities, such as shopping, food preparation, and cleaning. It's just not available, except from neighbors.

"The personal care facility is inadequate. There are a few nice rooms, but not many. That's why people wait so long before deciding to go to personal or nursing care. The home needs to have a better personal care facility, and maybe provide more services in the home."

The Working Session

Steve entered the final working session feeling confident in his recommendations, but uncertain about what the board's responses may be. Although committee members had talked freely during the interviews, they had been relatively quiet in the working sessions in which the analyses were presented. Steve did not know whether that was a positive sign or not. He had managed to raise a response from Mr. Polk on relatively minor points related to financial position. Steve assumed that he had done a thorough and professional job and took their silence to mean concurrence with his analyses. Steve presented the following options.

1. Basic option—no facility expansion

    a. Upgrade the financial management system especially the management of entrance fees and contingent liabilities for retirement village residents.

    b. Provide service contract options for retirement village residents which encourage continued independence. Such services may include transportation, on-site medical care, and housecleaning. Optional contracts would result in higher monthly fees to residents.

2. Expand and modernize current facilities

    a. Enlarge the Alzheimer's disease unit. This option would take advantage of the home's experience and allow for increased care of persons with later stages of the disease. It would also expand bed capacity and may ease problems with the waiting list.

    b. Expand and modernize the personal care unit. This is one of the most rapidly growing programs among continuing care retirement communities. The current units were found to be inadequate. Bathing facilities in particular need to be upgraded. An enhanced personal care unit may also make retirement living more attractive and result in growth in the retirement village. Replacement of the personal care rooms in the farmhouse may become necessary if the facility cannot continue to meet safety codes.

c. Develop master site plan for the retirement village. Growth has been unplanned to date. Future growth should be planned, including roads and sewage treatment plant improvements. Prospective residents should be given fewer options with new houses. The current system has discouraged sales in the past, especially to older persons who are not willing to expend the effort necessary to retain and supervise a builder.

In order to pursue this option, the board would need to hire an architect to layout alternatives and estimate costs. Financing arrangements will depend on the options selected. A total marketing effort should be embarked upon to support any program development effort.

3. Program Initiatives

a. Provide adult day care for persons with Alzheimer's disease. This has been identified as a need by the area agency on aging and the health systems agency. It could be done on-site and would complement the residential Alzheimer's unit. It would involve minimal investment.

Like previous meetings, few questions were raised. Mr. Polk disagreed that the current financial management system was inadequate. The other options appeared to be acceptable. Following this meeting the recommendations were to be presented to the board for approval and action.

At the conclusion of the meeting, Steve became uneasy. As he left for home, he wondered what went wrong. How could he further help the committee to decide or to take action? He couldn't help but think about Mr. Polk's faith in "seat of the pants" decisions. He had done the best job he could. He hoped to be able to assist the board in implementing the selected strategies. The waiting had begun.

Case 13

Conflicting Strategies for Market Expansion: Hospital-Based Home Health Services*

Carlos A. Muñoz

Carlos A. Muñoz, Ph.D. is Assistant Professor, Department Health Services Administration, School of Public Health, University of Puerto Rico.

The History of San Pablo Hospital

San Pablo Hospital is one of the largest investor-owned hospitals in Puerto Rico. It was founded in 1976 by a group of physicians for the express purpose of providing comprehensive, quality health services as determined by the needs of the community in its service area.

The original project consisted of 200 beds which was expanded in 1980 to 330 beds; the staff has grown to approximately 800 employees. As part of the original project, an adjacent office building was constructed by a sister corporation. A Family Medicine Center was organized in 1981 to provide comprehensive family health services, including rehabilitation care by a staff of board certified family physicians. This center also houses a residency program in family practice affiliated with the Caribbean Central University School of Medicine.

---

* This case is based on an actual facility but names, issues, and organizational responses were altered to raise points for teaching purposes.

San Pablo Hospital has experienced continuous growth in patient days. In fiscal year 1985, the hospital registered 96,340 patient days; this figure increased to 99,053 in fiscal year 1988. The average length of stay has also remained relatively constant, dropping from 5.8 to 5.5 days during the cited period. San Pablo recorded over 40,000 visits to the emergency department during fiscal year 1988. The hospital admitted 18,134 patients from a medical staff of 450 physicians divided between 191 active members with full privileges and 259 physicians with courtesy privileges. The San Pablo faculty is young; 40 percent of all admissions where made by physicians between 30-40 years of age. The 41-50 year-old group accounted for 29 percent of the admissions and the 51-60-year old group admitted another 25 percent. Physicians 61 years old or older admitted only 1 percent of all hospital admissions.

In 1984, a diagnostic imaging center was inaugurated offering three diagnostic modalities in radiological science: computerized axial tomography, nuclear medicine and ultrasonography. The imaging center operates 24 hours a day, seven days a week, and provides continuous service to both the hospital and nearby health care facilities, evenings and weekends.

The San Pablo Institute started operations in 1987. It provides ambulatory surgery services and houses the Family Medicine Center. In addition, the institute provides office space for a substantial number of physicians. The newest service expansion is the creation of a cardiovascular unit. The unit contains an invasive cardiovascular laboratory and cardiovascular surgery services. It is affiliated with the Texas Heart Institute and staffed by physicians with practices both in Houston and Puerto Rico.

As a result of these expansions, San Pablo Hospital has developed a standard among its peers in the provision of the most technologically advanced health care service available in the hospital industry. Furthermore, over the years, San Pablo Hospital demonstrated its capacity and commitment to expand and adapt to new market opportunities.

Surrounding Areas

A San Pablo patient origin study revealed there are 13 towns comprising its primary and secondary service areas with a population of 1,013,719. This population represents almost one-third of the total population of Puerto Rico. According to projections from the

Commonwealth of Puerto Rico Planning Board, by 1990 the population of these areas will grow approximately 18 percent to 1,185,000. Five other hospitals serve this area, three of which are privately owned and two operated by the government. The government hospitals mainly serve the uninsured population which accounts for approximately 50 percent of the total population in the area.

A study by the U.S. Census Bureau on commuting patterns of the population in the market area served by San Pablo Hospital indicates that the majority of people living in the service area also work within it. Towns neighboring Bayamon, where San Pablo Hospital is located, have a large concentration of manufacturing firms. In August 1988, the total civilian labor force for the service area was approximately 500,000 people with an unemployment rate of 10 percent which is below the 15 percent rate for the rest of the Island.

San Pablo Hospital enjoys a good reputation in the community, not only in Bayamon, but also in its surrounding towns. Activities, such as educational courses and conferences, one-day clinics, and children's vaccinations are given throughout the year at the hospital and in other locations such as shopping centers and elderly communities.

The Management Structure

San Pablo Hospital is headed by the board of directors composed of ten members, all of whom are stockholders of the corporation. The board delegates to its executive committee the power to make decisions whenever prompt measures need to be implemented. The executive committee consists of the chairperson, the president, the vice-president, the secretary, and the treasurer.

The board has designated an executive administrator and an executive medical director with the responsibility for administrative and medical affairs. The executive medical director deals directly with the medical affairs of the hospital. The clinical department heads report to the executive medical director. The executive administrator is accountable for the administrative affairs of the hospital. His staff is composed of two associate administrators, and the directors of finance, nursing services, engineering, human resources, and marketing. It is important to stress that this management team has been characterized by its low turnover rate. The executive administrator has occupied the position for the last eight years and has actively participated in the growth of the institution.

Caribbean Hospital Affiliates (CHA)

Created by San Pablo's directors, Caribbean Hospital Affiliates is a health care management company organized under the laws of the Commonwealth of Puerto Rico. Its primary objective is to offer consultation on organization, planning, supervision, and administration of hospitals, skilled nursing facilities, and other health related organizations. At present, utilizing San Pablo management staff as consultants, CHA manages three acute care hospitals. All three institutions are privately owned and are undergoing strategic modifications in their activities and programs, through CHA management programs.

Analyzing the Home Health Care Market

A Task Force is Formed

As part of an evaluation process of new market opportunities, the board of directors identified various factors that could encourage expansion of new services. These included:

- An increasingly aging population
- Availability of new technology for home use
- An increase in Medicare admissions coupled with the advent of the prospective payment for Medicare patients
- Strong cultural affinity for health care provided at home.

San Pablo has an approved certificate of need for 80 skilled nursing beds. To ensure a continuum of care, the executive committee studied the feasibility of entering into the home health care market and commissioned a special task force with the responsibility of implementing the board's mandate. Specifically, this task force was directed to conduct a market analysis of home health services and gather the necessary information to present a Certificate of Need to the Secretary of Health.

The task force consisted of the assistant administrator in charge of the Ambulatory Surgery and Family Medicine Center, the social worker in charge of discharge planning, the hospital associate legal counsel and a consultant from the academic community. The task force organized its work in two areas; external and internal market conditions and the Certificate of Need process. The administrator and discharge planner worked in the first area and the legal counsel worked in the other. The consultant worked in both areas serving as the liaison between them.

The task force prepared a preliminary report for discussion. It included recommendations for the development of a home health services program as a revenue-producing activity and an assessment of the prospects for government approval of a Certificate of Need. On September 5, a meeting with the board was held where the preliminary report was discussed. Also invited to this meeting, by the executive committee, were the executive administrator, the two associate administrators and the financial director.

The Task Force Report

The task force began by stating four main reasons for entering the home health services market. These were to ensure a continuum of care, achieve internal control over the cost, quality, and access to this service, manage hospital length of stay, increase revenue. The report outlined how hospital based home health services have grown in the United States since 1983. This growth was the product of changes in the reimbursement system and the spread of cost containment policies by insurance carriers that encourage the use of alternatives to the hospital setting. Although historically, the Puerto Rico health system was not subject to such stringent policies, the recent advent of the prospective payment system and its impact on length of stay will have affect on the health insurance market.

The task force then presented its market analysis of home health services; external market conditions were presented first. According to data from the Department of Health, in July 1988, there were 45 Medicare-certified home health care agencies in Puerto Rico. This translated to a ratio of 1.62 hospitals for every home health agency. There were four hospital-based and 41 free-standing, community based home health care agencies. The San Pablo service area was served by seven free standing home health agencies.

The task force reported that during the last fiscal year, the home health care agencies in Puerto Rico received $14.9 million in Medicare reimbursements. The average reimbursement per visit was $41.57 but ranged from as low as $33 to as high as $60. Average reimbursement for hospital based programs was $50 per visit. During that year, the agencies reported 360,467 visits averaging approximately 667 visits per agency per month. The hospital based home health programs were reimbursed $2.0 million; one agency received $7.0 million in Medicare reimbursement which accounts for almost 50 percent of the total market.

San Pablo Hospital data indicate that there were 751 patients discharged to home care last year. Of these, Medicare patients discharged to home care totalled 667 or 15 percent of all Medicare patient discharges. Non-Medicare discharges to home care represented 0.65 percent of all non-Medicare patients discharged.

From January to July of this year, the Medicare discharges increased to 18 percent, although total discharges increased by a smaller proportion. Also, the discharges to home care from other patient groups increased to 0.7 percent in the same period.

Since total discharges for this year remained constant, the figure of 19,000 discharges for last year was used to project service volume. The only figures changed to reflect the present trend were the percent discharges to home care. The 19,000 discharges were divided into 4,500 Medicare and 13,500 discharges for the remaining patient groups. The task force report projected a total of 13,515 home care visits, using an industry-wide standard of 15 visits per patient. Revenues were projected at $675,750 during the first year with an average reimbursement of $50 per visit.

The discharge planner explained that the projected volume of services was conservative. She argued that there are currently 30 physicians who generate more than 65 percent of all referrals to home care. Others do not refer patients to home health care agencies because they lack trust in the quality of their (agencies) services and fear the possibility of losing patients to the system. She presented the results of a survey conducted among hospital physicians showing 25 more physicians, (15 percent of the active medical staff) were willing to begin referring their patients to home care if San Pablo Hospital provided the services. Also, she argued that there was a gap in the services provided by most of the home health agencies serving the hospital. Over 40 percent of the cases began receiving treatment after the third day of discharge. She found cases in which the patient received the first visit one-week after discharge. In addition, most home health agencies did not accept referrals on weekends, so any patient discharged on a Saturday or Sunday had to wait until Monday to contact the agency to begin receiving the service. She concluded her presentation stating that if the hospital controlled this level of care it would enhance its image by extending the quality of its services to the patient's home. She was sure that more physicians would start referring to home care if the hospital was directly involved in the provision of the services.

Another member of the task force, the assistant administrator, explained that he was convinced home health services provided a good opportunity for hospital expansion. The hospital would extend the logical flow of referrals from both inpatient and outpatient settings to the patient's home. He added that this analysis focused only on one segment of the home care services market: skilled care. Additional opportunities existed in the durable medical equipment (DME) market and the use of the hospital's pharmacy to fill prescriptions directly in the patient's home.

The legal counsel presented an environmental assessment for Certificate of Need approval. He confirmed that home health care was regulated by Certificate of Need legislation established in 1975. The application process would require:

1. Notification of the hospital's intentions to the Secretary of Health 30 days before submitting an application.

2. After submitting the application, the hospital would have 30 days to submit additional information required by the Secretary of Health.

3. In the following 30-day period, the Secretary would notify all persons and entities affected by the application, and public notice would be published in the newspapers.

4. The application would then be evaluated by officials in the Department of Health. The evaluation process would consist of public hearings and evaluation of the proposals according to criteria established by the Department of Health.

The legal counsel noted that Department of Health standards for home health services included:

1. The geographic areas of service must coincide with one of the Department of Health's service areas.

2. No more than one home health agency for every 6,000 persons over age 65 in the proposed service area.

3. New agencies would not be approved until existing ones reached a total of 500 patients visits annually.

In his judgement, of the two quantitative standards for home care, one was met and the other possibily was met. He explained that San Pablo Hospital was within the Bayamon Health Region which was composed of 13 towns that were almost identical to the hospital's primary and secondary service areas. According to projections from the planning board, the area had a population of approximately 45,000 persons over 65 years old and was served by seven free-standing home health agencies. This meant there was an agency for every 6,400 persons over 65 years old living in this area. He argued that this distribution made the new service a borderline case for approval and that other arguments such as quality of care and the guarantee of the patients health care needs would have to be used to support the case. He did not visualize any problems about the third standard, because each of the seven agencies experienced an average of 700 patients per year.

He conceded that Department of Health officials were reluctant to grant any additional certificates of need for home health services in this area. He also expected strong opposition from the home health agencies serving the area. The legal counsel concluded by stating that San Pablo Hospital had faced stiffer battles for Certificate of Need approval and won; he cited the example of the Imaging Center. He stated emphatically that, although it could take at least a year, he was confident of approval of the hospital to provide home health services.

A Conflicting Vision

After the task force report was presented, the executive administrator felt that before any recommendations could be made to establish a hospital based home health services program, the board had to consider additional factors. First, he reminded the group that the Family Medicine Center and Caribbean Hospital Affiliates (CHA), the management and consulting company, were not fulfilling expectations for profitability. He added that the management company was supported not only with revenues generated from hospital services, but with management staff drawn away from the hospital to serve as CHA consultants, thereby impinging the normal flow of hospital operations.

He argued that these diversification efforts had not been as successful as projected and insisted that instead of venturing again into unknown prospects, it was time to solidify the hospital, the flagship of the system. The executive administrator stressed that San Pablo Hospital had been very successful because it had always been recognized as the most technologically advanced hospital in Puerto Rico and the Caribbean. He cited the positive example of the new cardiovascular unit which performs several unique diagnostic and surgical procedures and so ensures the hospital a competitive advantage over all other hospitals in Puerto Rico. He added that the cardiovascular unit had increased hospital revenues by 15 percent over the same period a year earlier. The expansion to other markets, he concluded, must be in the direction of establishing technologically advanced diagnostic and surgical procedures where he was convinced the competitive advantage of the hospital lay.

One of the associate administrators expressed concern about the home health services recommendations, stating that one hospital managed by CHA operated a home health service and its productivity left much to be desired. Whereas gross revenues amounted to $1 million, net losses totalled $200,000 a year. He attributed the losses to new Medicare reimbursement constraints and increased competition. Competition, he added, affected the hospital's revenue base. When hospital discharges were insufficient, other hospitals were not willing to refer patients to the CHA managed home health program fearing loss of patients to CHA.

While agreeing with the executive administrator's view, the associate administrator also supported the use of more home health services by hospital patients. With an effective case management program, the San Pablo Hospital could reduce Medicare patient lengths of stay and continue the health care process at home. In this manner, the hospital would maximize diagnostic-related group (DRG) reimbursement without having to undertake the responsibility of a home health care operation. He felt that this service would increase administrative and operational costs and increase malpractice insurance premiums.

The associate administrator's views brought focus to additiononal risk factors that would have to be considered by the institution including transportation problems; staff injuries; treatment errors; exposure to combative patients and high-risk neighborhoods; patient emergencies when staff members are not present; and personal losses reported by patient or family members during or after staff members visit to the patient's home. He concluded his critique by questioning whether it was worth engaging in a lengthy Certificate of Need approval process when the returns of the proposed home health services venture were uncertain.

The Task Force Reply

The assistant administrator stated that these last arguments were not based on detailed information about the operation of hospital-based home health services. He went on to explain that the task force analyzed the operations of the CHA hospital home health services program mentioned by the associate administrator and found two leading causes that produced the losses. The first was nursing productivity. A staff of 18 full-time nurses averaged 1.5 visits per day. Even when demand was low, the number of positions could not be reduced due to the collective bargaining agreements with the General Workers Union. A second problem was the Medicare claims denial rate. The home health program was experiencing a claims denial rate of almost ten percent, which was extremely high compared to industry standards. The denial rate resulted from an absence of training for the nurses in Medicare procedures and morale problems.

The assistant administrator felt that the CHA hospital-based home care program experienced management problems, not market problems as the associate administrator had insisted. Also, he reminded board members that San Pablo workers had consistently rejected all organizing initiatives by labor unions. This allowed for staffing flexibility within the proposed home health services geared to demand and permitted the establishment of staff productivity standards.

Regarding the issue of increased operational cost, the assistant administrator also reported that hospital-based home care programs received added reimbursement to cover higher administrative and general costs than do free-standing, community-based home health agencies. Allocations of some overhead costs could be shifted from the hospital to the home care department. He insisted that hospital-based home health programs provide advantages in access to patients, physicians, and hospital resources such as finance, health records, data processing, and risk management.

The Board's Reaction

After discussing the merits of the issues presented, the board decided more information was necessary before adopting a strategy. The chairman asked members of the task force to present more data on the implementation and operation of the program. Then, the executive administrator was commissioned to transform his vision of market expansion into specific projects. He was asked to submit a program of projects supported with data on their market potentials. The meeting was adjourned with agreement to continue the discussion within three weeks.

Case 14

A Contractual Tightrope:
Sunny Acres Villa, Inc.*

Heidi Boerstler

Heidi Boerstler, Dr. P.H., is Assistant Professor, School of Nursing, College of Business and Administration, University of Colorado.

Sunny Acres Villa, Inc. is a large, nonprofit, lifecare organization headquartered in Denver, Colorado. In 1969, when Sunny Acres began, it offered the elderly 175 apartments and 60 nursing home beds. In 1989, it offered 720 apartments, 182 nursing home beds, and 39 personal care beds. In the interim, it has also joined the Sisters of Charity Health Care Systems—the tenth largest chain of health facilities in the United States. Despite this growth, the Sunny Acres facility still faces complex problems involving admission standards, occupancy rates, corporate policies, and ambiguous demographic trends. The continued success of the facility appears to rest on board room decisions and the ability of its management to untangle policy and program issues.

The Life-Care Concept

Perhaps the most critical health policy issue facing the nation in the decades ahead is providing for the needs of the elderly. At mid-century, persons over age 65 years represented about 10 percent

---

* This is a true case based on issues confronting Sunny Acres Villa management and staff. Fictitious names of both the organization and individuals are used to ensure anonymity.

of the U.S. population; by the year 2000, they will represent 15 percent or more. And, persons over age 85, the persons with the highest need for health and social services, comprise the fastest growing segment of the U.S. population. With more elderly to provide for, more rational ways of providing for their long-term health and social and housing needs must be found. One option which is gaining popularity with policy makers is the life care community.

A life care community is a facility or cluster of facilities that offers independent living units—apartments, rooms, or cottages—and guarantees a range of health and social services, such as homemaker and skilled nursing care, to the residents in exchange for prepaid fees. In most instances, there are two types of fees: an entry fee (a substantial amount), which is paid before the person becomes a resident of the community; and a monthly fee (usually a modest amount), paid after the person becomes a resident. At Sunny Acres, the entry fee is $50,000 and the monthly fee is about $750.

The relationship between the life care community and the resident is contractual, and most often covers the remaining years of the resident's life. The contract defines the service obligations of the life care community and the financial obligations of the resident.

Life care is an attractive option to many elderly. It guarantees nursing care, housing, and other services for their remaining years, and alleviates many of their financial anxieties about paying for the services.

The Sunny Acres' mission statement reflects the philosophy of many life care communities.

Mission Statement

We at Sunny Acres believe . . . an elder is a person who is still developing, still growing, still a learner, still with potential, whose life continues to have within it promise for and connections to the future. Therefore, we are dedicated to:

Provide innovative support services and personal growth opportunities which promote the physical . . . financial . . . emotional . . . social . . . and spiritual well-being and meet changing needs of individuals age 62 and older.

Be open and responsive to our residents.

Provide enriching employment opportunities which will influence staff and resident commonality of purpose.

Extend our leadership in providing quality residential and health care services to others outside our life-care communities.

The History of Sunny Acres

When Sunny Acres incorporated in October 1969, it consisted of one 175-apartment living center and one 60-bed nursing center; within three years, additional facilities were purchased in Colorado Springs (in 1969) and Pueblo (in 1971). By 1976, Sunny Acres had reached its current capacity of 720 apartments, of which 372 are located in Denver, 202 are in two facilities in Colorado Springs, and 146 are in Pueblo. Nursing home beds also increased to 182 with 118 in Denver and 32 each in Colorado Springs and Pueblo. In addition, each Sunny Acres community also has between 12 and 14 personal care beds for residents no longer able to manage in their apartments but who do not require continuous skilled nursing services. (Table 14-1)

Last May, Sunny Acres broke ground for a new 90-bed nursing facility at the Pueblo community. Current plans for the facility include 59 skilled nursing beds and 31 personal care beds; the $4 million project is scheduled for completion next year.

Table 14-1 Sunny Acres Villa, Inc. organizational chart.

	Denver	Colorado Springs	Pueblo	Total
Apartment units	372	202	146	720
Nursing home beds	118	32	32	182
Personal care beds	12	13	14	39

Sisters of Charity Affiliation

For most of its existence, Sunny Acres has weathered financial difficulties in a resolute struggle to survive. In 1986, the board of directors approved what appeared to be a mutually beneficial affiliation with the Sisters of Charity Health Care Systems, Inc., in Cincinnati, Ohio. Sisters of Charity, a large, multihospital system, wanted to expand its services to the elderly, and the Sunny Acres board of directors welcomed the strengthened financial position offered by the major health care system.

As a result of the affiliation, Sunny Acres also created a for-profit subsidiary, Centennial Management, Inc., to provide consulting and management expertise in retirement housing and elderly health care services, primarily to other members of the Sisters of Charity system. Currently, Centennial has management contracts with several other Sisters' affiliates.

Advantages to Affiliation

The Sunny Acres' chief executive officer saw two strong advantages to the Sisters of Charity affiliation:

> First, Sunny Acres has better access to capital, at better terms, than it had without the affiliation. Most life care communities, for example, are unrated for purposes of issuing debt; Sisters of Charity has an A++ debt rating, which improves Sunny Acres' ability to borrow.

> Second, the Sisters of Charity affiliation gives Sunny Acres access to lower cost group insurance programs, including the bane of all health-care programs, liability insurance. Also, the Sisters of Charity system guarantees all resident contracts. For example, if the Colorado insurance commissioner quashed the sale of life care contracts, Sisters of Charity would be required to support Sunny Acres until the final existing contract had run its course.

However, because Sisters of Charity bears much of the Sunny Acres' financial responsibility, it maintains considerable fiscal control over them. Sisters sets limits on the amount of debt Sunny Acres may carry and has authority over dissolution of assets and board membership; it also has the final word on the Sunny Acres' budget.

Corporate Structure

Board of Directors

The Sunny Acres' board of directors is made up of 20 members; under terms of the affiliation, it includes representatives from each of its three life care communities, local business persons, and representatives of the Sisters of Charity Health Care System. It has five standing committees—marketing, finance, building, quality assurance, and nominating and policy—and meets six times per year. Of the 20 members, six seats are held by the Sisters of Charity system.

The Management Team

Sunny Acres' executive management team includes the corporation's president and chief executive officer, chief financial officer, director of marketing, executive directors of the three Sunny Acres communities, and Centennial Management's chief operating officer (Exhibit 14-1).

Resident Profile and Options

Demographics

Although the youngest age for a person to qualify for Sunny Acres' residency is 62 years, the typical new resident is age 76. New residents have average assets of about $150,000 and monthly incomes of $2,000 to $2,500. Eighty-five percent of them come from Colorado, predominantly from the Denver area (Table 14-2). Generally, they purchase one-bedroom apartments with life-care contracts, pay entry fees of $50,000, and pay monthly service fees of $750. The average length of time they remain in the life-care community is 13 years. (This compares with two to three years for so-called senior apartment residents, 18 to 24 months for nursing-home residents, and only three to four days for hospital patients.)

Self-Selection

It is important to recognize that residents of a life-care community are a highly self-selected population; that is, they specifically

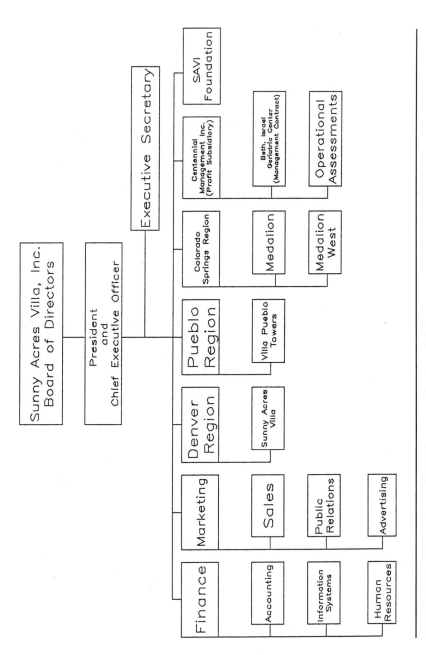

Exhibit 14-1 Sunny Acres Villa, Inc. organizational chart.

Table 14-2 New residents demographics (June 1, 1983 through May 31, 1985).

Characteristic	Number	Percent
Home of origin		
25 miles	82	55%
Colorado	26	17%
Out of state	41	28%
Total	149	100%
Lead source		
Yellow Pages	8	5%
Direct mail	4	3%
Newspaper	18	12%
Magazine	8	5%
Resident referral	33	22%
Referral	67	45%
Other source	11	8%
Total	149	100%
Months: Initial contact to occupancy		
Under 1 year	128	86%
1-2 years	19	13%
Over 2 years	2	1%
Total	149	100%
Marital status		
Single	107	72%
Couple	42	28%
Total	149	100%
Apartment type		
Studio	43	29%
1 Bedroom	67	45%
1 Bedroom Combo	4	3%
2 Bedroom	35	23%
Total	149	100%
Facility		
Sunny Acres Villa	81	54%
Medalion	16	11%
Medalion West	24	16%
Villa Pueblo	28	19%
Total	149	100%
Sex		
Male	61	32%
Female	130	68%
Total	191	100%

and deliberately chose this particular retirement lifestyle. There fore, as a group, they share many more attitudes, habits, and social characteristics among themselves than they share with the population as a whole. Significant indicators of their self-selection, all of which influence the management and operation of the life-care community, include:

Residency Choice. Residents choose, while still functionally able to make choices, to live in a life care community; a rather large segment of the U.S. population likely would not make such a choice.

Economic Status. Residents are better off financially than the average person their age. Among other things, this indicates that their working years were more prosperous, if not more satisfying, than most of their peers and that they have developed a regard for the accumulation of assets.

Residency Commitment. Residents tend to make life-long commitments to remain in the life care community—commitments that include a high level of interest in, and concern over, community management decisions.

Community Involvement. Life care residents tend to be advocates for themselves and other residents and often form and actively participate in resident associations (more similar to homeowner or tenant associations than to "sunshine clubs").

Functional Longevity. Life care residents maintain functional independence longer than most elderly patients. They are, therefore, more capable of understanding current events and of developing and articulating opinions than are many persons of similar age.

Financial Interest. Residents clearly have a financial interest in the management decisions of their life care communities. They pay for their services and care out of their own pockets, most often making an initial investment in excess of $50,000. And most are aware that, in the past, some life care communities have undergone bankruptcy.

Contractual Arrangements

Sunny Acres offers prospective residents three contract options: traditional life care, monthly residency, and capital refund. The monthly residency and capital refund programs are designed to increase occupancy by attracting persons who may be wary of, or uncertain about, the life care concept.

Traditional Life Care. The Sunny Acres' traditional life care contract can take any of several variations, but basically it entitles purchasers to resident and nursing care for the remainder of their lifetimes in exchange for entry and monthly fees (Exhibit 14-2).

Monthly Residency. In addition to the life care contract, Sunny Acres offers a monthly program in which residents pay monthly fees but no entry fee. They enjoy Sunny Acres' health care services, nursing care, home care, medications, dietary and recreational programs—all conveniently located on campus—but are only available on a fee-for-service basis.

Capital Refund. The capital refund program is similar to the traditional life care program except that when a resident dies or leaves Sunny Acres, 90 percent of the entry fee is refunded; however, the entry fee is 50 percent higher than that of the traditional program.

Admission to Sunny Acres

A person accepted for Sunny Acres' residency must be at least 62 years of age (younger spouses may enter, of course, but they must also pay a premium). The applicant must also be able to live independently when first entering the community.

Admission to Sunny Acres is admission for life. A careful and critical assessment of each applicant, therefore, is crucial, mainly for Sunny Acres' risk management strategies; consequently, the admission process is often lengthy, involving financial, health, and social services assessments (Exhibit 14-3).

Financial Assessment. An applicant undergoes a financial assessment to determine his or her ability to pay the initial entry and monthly service fees. Assuming the applicant clears the financial hurdle, he or she is given a two-part medical assessment and a social services assessment.

Physician Assessment. A person's ability to live independently is judged in several ways, but basically applicants submit to physical examinations by their personal physicians to determine if they have physical problems that could interfere with independent living.

SUNNY ACRES VILLA, INC.

RESIDENCY AGREEMENT

I. PARTIES TO THIS AGREEMENT

A. The parties to this Agreement are a facility of Sunny Acres Villa, Inc., hereinafter called Community, and _____, hereinafter designated as Resident. (Community refers jointly to the facility and the corporation. If two (2) persons sign this Residency Agreement, Resident refers to and shall apply to both persons, unless specifically stated otherwise in this Agreement.)

B. Sunny Acres Villa, Inc., a nonprofit life care corporation licensed by the State of Colorado, has its principal place of business at 2501 E. 104th Avenue, Thornton, Colorado, 80233.

C. Benefits offered under the terms of this Agreement are nontransferable and shall automatically terminate upon the death of the Resident.

II. OBLIGATIONS OF THE COMMUNITY

A. In consideration of payment of the entry fee and monthly service fee as established in Section IV, the Community shall provide the following services at no additional charge to the Resident:

1. Unfurnished living accommodations to the Resident for life in the Community subject to existing licensure laws, termination and transfer as provided in this Agreement.
2. Unlimited days of nursing care per person in the licensed health care center. The rates charged for health center care are specified in Section VI, D.
3. Carpeting, refrigerator, range and garbage disposal in all apartment units.
4. Electricity, heat, water, sewer and garbage removal.
5. Limited services by nursing personnel in the Resident's apartment to assist the Resident with his/her home health needs.
6. The monitoring of a 24-hour emergency call system by nursing personnel.
7. All regular and necessary maintenance, repairs and replacement of Community property.
8. Redecoration of living unit in accordance with policy established by the Community's Board of Directors.
9. Groundskeeping.
10. Bi-weekly general housekeeping services.
11. Periodic cleaning of windows, carpets and Community property.
12. Bi-weekly flat laundry services for sheets, pillow cases, towels and washcloths.
13. Limited or regularly-scheduled transportation to and from some local businesses, neighborhood churches, local shopping centers and local medical facilities (non-emergency).
14. Security systems and staff for the protection of the Resident. The community does not, however, assume responsibility for loss or damage suffered by the resident.

June, 1984 Residency Agreement

Exhibit 14-2 Residency agreement Sunny Acres Villa.

15. A centrally located mail distribution system.
16. The availability of an activity program to stimulate the Residents mentally, socially and physically.
17. One parking spot per unit for those having automobiles.
18. The service of a chaplain who shall conduct or coordinate nondenominational worship service and Bible studies.

B. Services for which the Resident is charged in addition to the entry fee and monthly service fee:

1. The Community shall provide dining facilities, where meals may be purchased by the Resident. An extra charge shall be made for tray service to individual apartments as approved by the Community for health reasons and for special diets. Guest meals shall be available for a charge and may be arranged for through the food service department.
2. While the Resident is a patient in the health care center state health department regulations require the Community to provide three (3) meals per day, for which the Resident will be charged. Certain other services may be charged as specified in Section VI, C.
3. The Community charges the Resident for medical supplies and appliances and for some treatments and services provided in the Resident's apartment.
4. At the Resident's expense, optional redecoration or redecoration done more frequently than established by policy may be done upon approval of the Community.
5. Housekeeping services beyond those normally provided or services requested more frequently than biweekly are available at prevailing rates and as previously authorized by the Community.
6. The Community shall provide laundry machines and facilities for the use by Residents at their own expense.
7. The Community shall provide guest apartments for a charge when available, upon advance registration through the business office.
8. Special transportation beyond that normally provided without charge may be made available by the Community at a reasonable charge.
9. The Community may provide shopping service at prevailing rates upon prior approval of the Community.
10. The Community may establish reasonable rates for garages, if available.
11. Unless specifically stated in this Agreement, other services are not normally provided by the Community, but may be provided at the Resident's expense.

III. OBLIGATIONS OF THE RESIDENT

A. Whereas the primary objective of the Community is to create an environment of well-being for the Resident, each Resident has the responsibility and is expected to make all reasonable efforts to be agreeable to other Residents and to cooperate with the management of the Community in maintaining a pleasant and harmonious environment at all times.

June, 1984 Residency Agreement

Exhibit 14-2, continued.

B. The Resident shall be responsible for the payment of the entry fee, monthly service fee, meal charges, charges for noncovered items and services specified in Section VI, C and other such miscellaneous fees as are provided under this Agreement.

C. The Resident shall meet his/her financial responsibilities to the Community and shall advise the Community of any change in the Resident's financial condition which might affect the ability to meet his/her financial responsibilities to the Community.

D. In the event the Resident intentionally divests his/her financial resources to the extent that the Resident is unable to meet the financial requirements of this Agreement, such divestiture shall constitute a breach of this Agreement, and the Community shall be entitled to dismiss the Resident in accordance with the provisions of Section VIII, C.

E. The Resident shall not alter or cause to be altered any structural part of his/her apartment or any permanently installed feature thereof, without the written permission of the administrator of the Community. If permitted, such alteration shall conform to acceptable standards required by the Community.

F. The Resident shall file a confidential statement on a form supplied by the Community, designating the person(s) who is authorized to act on his/her behalf and to enter the Resident's apartment in the event of the Resident's disability or death and shall keep the confidential statement current. The Community encourages the Resident to execute a will and to file a statement with the Community's business office as to who has a copy of that will. In addition, the Resident shall grant the Community the right of entry into the Resident's apartment in the case of an emergency or by special request at reasonable hours. The intent of this provision is to assure that the Community complies with the Resident's intentions, to authorize the Community to relate with such designated individual(s) and to maintain security of the Resident's apartment in emergency situations.

G. The Resident is responsible for his/her personal telephone bill.

H. The Resident is liable for any loss, damage or expense suffered by the Community as a result of negligence by the Resident.

I. The Community does not insure the personal property of residents. The Resident is responsible for losses to the Resident's personal property. The Community encourages Residents to carry their own liability insurance coverage and such fire, theft, and comprehensive coverage as may be necessary to provide adequate coverage on their property.

J. The Resident agrees to abide by any written rules or procedures of the Community.

K. Pets are permitted only when the Community expressly agrees to such in writing. Generally, pets such as cats and dogs are permitted only in cottage units.

June, 1984 Residency Agreement

Exhibit 14-2, continued.

L. If the Resident desires to change his/her residency status, except for termination, such change must receive the prior approval of the Community. This provision includes, but is not limited to, changes in residency status which occur because of transfer to another apartment and joint residency arrangements.

M. The Resident shall carry an insurance policy covering hospitalization and medical expenses, either through Medicare and supplemental coverage or a private insurance contract with equivalent coverage.

IV. FEES

A. Entry Fee:
1. The Resident shall pay the Community an entry fee of $_____ for apartment #_____.

2. Payment shall be made as follows:_____

_____

_____

B. Monthly Service Fee:

1. A monthly service fee, due and payable in advance by the Resident on the first day of each month, is now set at $_____ per month.
2. The Community may adjust the monthly service fee as determined necessary by the Board of Directors.
3. The Community shall provide the Resident with thirty (30) days written notice before adjusting the monthly service fee.
4. When the Resident is away from the Community for any length of time, no credit on the monthly service fee is given to the Resident.

V. REFUND OF ENTRY FEE

A. If this Agreement is terminated within allowable limits following the date of this Agreement, the Resident shall receive a partial refund of the entry fee. The amount of the refund shall be determined by the following formula and shall be paid subject to the provisions in paragraph B below:

1. Within sixty (60) days following the date of this Agreement, the Resident or the Community may exercise the right to rescind this Agreement by notifying the other party in writing and, by so doing, the Resident shall be entitled a full refund of the entry fee paid to the Community.
2. If termination occurs for reasons other than death after sixty (60) days, but within five (5) years following the date of this Agreement, the Resident shall receive a refund equal to the entry fee paid: (1) less the amount earned by the Community at the rate of one and

June, 1984 Residency Agreement

Exhibit 14-2, continued.

two-thirds (1.667) percent per month of occupancy; (2) less medical
expenses incurred by the Community on behalf of the Resident; and (3)
less amounts due from the Resident for damages done or any other
legitimate offsetting item.

B. The Community shall refund any and all monies due a former Resident or
his/her estate within thirty (30) days of closing on another Residency
Agreement for the vacated apartment. No interest shall be payable on any
refund provided for in this Agreement.

VI. HEALTH CARE SERVICES

A. The Community operates a licensed health care center for the benefit of the
Residents. Each Resident has unlimited lifetime nursing care in the
Community's health care center, which includes skilled, intermediate,
personal or clinic nursing care, at the level of need and in other than a
private room. If available, the Resident may request private accommodations
upon payment of an additional charge.

B. The Community maintains a licensed nursing staff to provide or supervise
limited nursing services in the Resident's apartment. These services are
provided at the discretion of the Community and may be provided at
additional charge to the Resident.

C. Although the provisions of this Agreement provide many health care services
to the Resident, either in the licensed health care center or the Resident's
apartment, there are services that are not provided the Resident, or if
provided, are provided at the Resident's expense:

1. State health department regulations require the Community's health care
center to provide three (3) meals per day to patients. Residents
admitted on either a temporary or permanent basis to the health care
center shall be charged for meal service.
2. All medicines and drugs, medical supplies and appliances, special health
care and treatments, if provided, are provided at the Resident's
expense.
3. Hospitalization, physician services and emergency transportation are not
provided under this Agreement. The Resident may use the physician of
his/her choice, it being expressly understood that the Resident is
responsible for payment of any physician charges. In an emergency, the
Community is authorized to seek at Resident's expense the assistance of
a licensed health care practitioner if the Resident's personal physician
cannot be reached.
4. The Community is licensed to provide skilled and intermediate nursing
care. This Agreement does not obligate the Community to provide housing
or services beyond the scope of those authorized by licensure. Examples
of services which the Community does not provide are psychiatric care,
drug rehabilitation and treatment, care for contagious diseases, and
acute hospitalization care.

June, 1984 Residency Agreement

Exhibit 14-2, continued.

D. Charges to the Resident assigned either temporarily or permanently to the Community's health care center shall be as follows:

   1. Monthly Service Fee

      a. In the case of retention of apartment - If the apartment occupied by the Resident is retained for the use by a Resident temporarily assigned to the health care center or by a joint Resident of a Resident permanently assigned to the health care center, the Resident's monthly service fee shall remain the same.

      b. In the case of relinquishment of apartment - If the apartment occupied by the Resident is relinquished to the Community upon the Resident's permanent assignment to the health care center, the Resident's monthly service fee shall be based on the monthly service fee for the Community's most common studio apartment.

   2. Credit for Medicare Payment

   The Community shall credit the Resident for Medicare payment for meals or items and services provided the Resident at an additional charge while the Resident is assigned to the health care center. All Medicare payments otherwise become the property of the Community.

VII. RELINQUISHMENT OF ACCOMMODATIONS

A. The Resident may choose to move out of his/her apartment unit at any time, by giving sixty (60) days advance written notice and shall receive a refund of the entry fee as provided in Section V. The Resident shall be responsible to pay the applicable monthly service fee during the sixty (60) day notification period.

B. If a Resident is unable to live independently, the Community may transfer him/her to an accommodation providing the services needed by the Resident. After ninety (90) days continuous assignment to the Community's health care center or a hospital, the Community may initiate consideration of a permanent transfer and if so determined, may require the Resident to relinquish the apartment unit. The determination of such a permanent transfer is done jointly with the Resident, the attending physician, the Community's administrator and the Community's medical director, if needed, and any others who may be appropriate, including the Resident's family. The purpose of the joint decision-making process is to make the best determination for the Resident under the given circumstances. The ultimate authority in this process is the Community.

C. If it is later determined that the Resident's condition has improved to such an extent that he/she is capable of resuming independent living, the Community shall offer the apartment relinquished by the Resident or, if that apartment is unavailable, a similar apartment. The monthly service fee charged the Resident will be the current rate charged for the apartment occupied by the Resident.

June, 1984 Residency Agreement

Exhibit 14-2, continued.

D. If two persons occupy the same apartment and one dies or vacates the apartment, the remaining Resident shall be entitled to remain in sole possession and occupy said accommodation, and the monthly service fee shall be adjusted to reflect the single occupancy.

E. Removal of possessions - When the sole surviving Resident relinquishes an apartment, through death or otherwise, the Resident or the estate or representative of the Resident shall be responsible for the removal of all personal property from the Community. The Resident or Resident's estate shall be responsible for payment of all outstanding charges due the Community, including payment of the monthly service fee until the apartment is vacated. If the Resident's personal property has not been removed within ninety (90) days of relinquishing the apartment, the Community may remove and store personal property of the Resident at the expense of the Resident or Resident's estate. Only those individuals designated by the Resident in writing shall be granted access to the apartment by the Community.

VIII. MISCELLANEOUS PROVISIONS

A. Care and Removal of Mentally or Physically Impaired Residents:

1. If, in the opinion of the Community's physician, any Resident should be placed in the health care center because of the Resident's mental or physical condition, the administrator of the local Community shall have the authority to take such steps as may be appropriate to accomplish the same, subject to the policies of the Community.

2. If any resident should not reside in the Community because of a mental or physical condition for which the Community is not authorized by license to provide care or which jeopardizes the health and safety of other residents or that of the Resident, the Community's Board of Directors, acting upon the recommendation of the Community's administrator and physician, the Resident, the attending physician and any others who may be appropriate, shall have the authority to take such steps as may be appropriate to have the Resident placed elsewhere for care at the Resident's expense. If this occurs, all obligations of the Community shall terminate, except that the Community shall pay to the Resident or to the legal representative or guardian of a mentally or physically ill Resident such refund as specified in Section V. If a Resident so removed from the Community later recovers to the extent he/she is able to return to the Community, as determined by the Community's physician and administrator, the Resident shall have restored all the rights and privileges of this Residency Agreement conditioned upon repayment of the refund, if any, of the entry fee made to the Resident at the time of removal from the Community.

B. Appointment of Guardian or Conservator - If any Resident becomes legally incompetent, a relative of that Resident, any person designated by the Resident in his/her personal file in the business office to act on behalf of the Resident or the administrator may file for the appointment of a guardian or conservator for the Resident.

June, 1984 Residency Agreement

Exhibit 14-2, continued.

C. Dismissal - Willful misrepresentation by any Resident of any material fact in Resident's application to the Community or any act or conduct by the Resident which, in the judgment of the Board of Directors, jeopardizes the welfare of the other Residents or interferes with proper administration of the Community shall be cause for termination by the Community of this Resident's Agreement and dismissal and removal of the Resident from the Community. Written notice of pending proceedings shall be given to the Resident involved by personal delivery or by certified postal delivery to the last known address. Any Resident for whom dismissal from the Community is under consideration shall have the right to appear before the Board of Directors, for a hearing with regard to the dismissal. The judgment of the Board of Directors at the conclusion of the hearing is final in all respects.

D. Validity of this Agreement - The invalidity of any restriction, condition or other provision of this Agreement, in whole or in part, shall not impair or affect in any way the validity, enforceability or effect of the remainder of this Agreement.

IX. SUBORDINATION

The Resident agrees that the rights of a lender under any deed of trust executed by the Community may now or in the future have priority over the rights of the Resident under this Agreement, except as provided by C.R.S. 12-13-106.

X. RIGHTS OF THE RESIDENT

A. The rights of the Resident under this Agreement are the rights and privileges herein expressly granted and do not include any proprietary interest in the properties or operations of the Community, and are subject to such subordination agreements as set forth in Section IX.

B. This Agreement and the Application for Residency contain the entire agreement between the parties, and no amendment or addendum of this Agreement or promise is valid or enforceable unless executed in writing and signed by the Resident and the Community.

C. The rights of the Resident under this Agreement do not confer any authority to any Resident, acting individually or collectively, to participate in the management of the Community. The Community encourages the Resident to participate in the activities of the residents' association, whose sole authority is advisory and whose constitution and bylaws are consistent with the bylaws of the Community's Board of Directors.

D. The Resident has the right to employ individuals to assist him/her in maintaining independent living; however, such right is secondary to the rights and interests of the Community and other residents. The Community has the right to prior authorization of live-in employment arrangements involving a Resident and to impose any charges to recover the costs incurred by the Community because of such employment. The Community may terminate or

June, 1984 Residency Agreement

Exhibit 14-2, continued.

impose conditions affecting the Resident's right to employ individuals in such capacity if the Resident or person employed violates the rules and procedures of the Community or acts in a manner inconsistent with the rights and interests of the Community and other residents.

XI. EFFECTIVE DATE OF AGREEMENT/OCCUPANCY

By mutual agreement and consent of the Community and the Resident(s) whose signatures appear below, the effective date of this Agreement hereinafter acknowledged as the date of occupancy shall be the _____ day of _____, 19__. The Resident hereby acknowledges receipt of the Community's most recent audited statements for the previous 24-month period ended _____.

SUNNY ACRES VILLA, INC.   RESIDENT(S)

_____   _____
Signature   Signature

                                           _____
                                           Signature

_____   _____
Date   Date

                                           SAVI 6-84

June, 1984 Residency Agreement

Exhibit 14-2, continued.

SUNNY ACRES VILLA, INC.

APPLICATION FOR RESIDENCY

I. PARTIES TO THE APPLICATION

   A. The parties to this application are _____,
a facility of Sunny Acres Villa, Inc., hereinafter called the Community,
and _____, hereinafter
designated as the Applicant. (Community refers jointly to the facility
and the corporation. If two persons sign this Application, the term
Applicant refers to both persons.)

   B. Sunny Acres Villa, Inc., a nonprofit life care corporation licensed by
the State of Colorado, has its principal place of business at 2501 E.
104th Avenue, Thornton, Colorado 80233.

II. ELIGIBILITY QUALIFICATIONS OF APPLICANT

   A. Age - Applicants shall be at least 62 years of age. When more than one
person becomes an Applicant, one must be at least age 62.

   B. Health Status - The Applicant shall submit a confidential medical report
prepared by his/her personal physical on forms supplied by the Community
as a part of this Application. The purpose of the medical report and any
tests or examinations related thereto is to:

      1. assist the Community in determining acceptability of the Applicant to
reside in the Community and to live in an independent environment;
      2. provide the Community with an initial health assessment on each
Applicant which will assist the Community in the appropriate delivery
of any future health care services, should the Applicant be approved
for residency.

The medical report shall be reviewed by the Community and the cost of any
tests or examinations required as a part of health status determinations
shall be the responsibility of the Applicant.

   C. Financial Ability - The Applicant shall submit a confidential financial
report on forms supplied by the Community as a part of this Application.
The purpose of the financial report is to assist the Community in
determining whether the Applicant would be able to meet the financial
obligations of residency in the Community. The Applicant hereby
authorizes the Community to make such investigations and contact any
person to verify the financial information indicated by the Applicant on
the submitted report. The Resident shall carry an insurance policy
covering hospitalization and medical expenses, either through Medicare
and supplemental coverage or a private insurance contract with equivalent
coverage.

Exhibit 14-3 Application for residency Sunny Acres Villa.

D. Sociability - The Applicant may be required to submit a confidential report on forms supplied by the Community and submit references of individuals who can attest to the Applicant's personal habits, lifestyle and disposition toward other persons as a part of this Application. The purpose of this review is to assist the Community in bringing into residency those who will be compatible, and not unreasonably objectionable, to other residents.

E. Persons not deranged in mind nor afflicted with any contagious, infectious, or mental disease, nor any other disease or condition considered by the Community to be objectionable, will be considered for residency in the Community. Applicants shall be considered for residency regardless of race, color, religion, national origin, sex, age or handicap, provided such handicap does not interfere with the Applicant's ability to live independently.

F. NO APPLICANT SHALL BE ACCEPTED FOR RESIDENCY IN THE COMMUNITY UNTIL THE COMMUNITY HAS APPROVED IN WRITING THAT THE APPLICANT HAS MET AGE, HEALTH STATUS, FINANCIAL ABILITY AND SOCIABILITY STANDARDS.

III. RESERVATION OF APARTMENT - DEPOSIT REQUIRED

A. The Community agrees to reserve Apartment _____ located at

_____ for
(Community)   (Street Address)   (City and State)

the Applicant upon payment of the deposit of $_____, which Community hereby acknowledges receipt and which shall apply toward the full entry fee of $_____, until the scheduled date of residency, which shall be _____.

B. In the case of two Applicants in which one is below the minimum age, the Community shall assess an additional charge based upon the Applicant's age as of the effective date of the Residency Agreement.

C. The Community agrees to hold in escrow the deposited money until the effective date of the Residency Agreement as required by state law.

D. It is expressly understood by both parties that the Community does not pay interest on any deposit.

Exhibit 14-3, continued.

E. The Applicant shall make a good faith effort to assume residency on the date indicated in paragraph A above. If Applicant later determines that he/she will be unable to assume residency by the established date, the Applicant hereby agrees to relinquish the reservation of the living unit indicated in paragraph A above. The Community, in its sole discretion, may extend or renew this Application beyond the date specified, may elect to require the Applicant to reapply, or may elect to accept the Applicant for residency upon execution of a secured instrument and payment of fees customary to residency in the Community.

F. With the exception of reserving the apartment specified in paragraph A above, this Application shall not give the Applicant any of the privileges or rights granted residents of the Community.

IV. REFUND OF DEPOSIT

A. If the Applicant should decide for any reason to withdraw this Application, the Community shall refund to the Applicant any and all funds deposited by the Applicant with the Community. No interest is payable by the Community on such deposit.

B. A request for refund by the Applicant shall be in writing to the Community.

C. Any refund of the deposit requested by the Applicant shall be payable by the Community within thirty (30) days of the Community's receipt of such request.

D. The Community is required by state law to provide the Applicant with the most recent two (2) years' audited financial statements of the corporation prior to residency, for which the Applicant hereby acknowledges receipt.

_____
Applicant

Executed this____day of_____, 19__.

Applicant(s)   Applicant(s) address

_____   _____

Signature   _____

_____

Signature

The Community hereby certifies that the Applicant has met the requirements for residency, including age, health, financial and sociability standards, this _____ day of_____, 19__.

_____

Administrator

Exhibit 14-3, continued.

Nursing Assessment. In addition to a medical assessment, each Sunny Acres community conducts its own nursing assessment of each applicant. In theory, the nursing assessment projects the applicant's present and future nursing need and demand. It includes evaluations of both physical ability (primarily for daily living activities) and functional or mental status (such as the presence or absence of confusion and disorientation) to determine the applicant's ability to live independently.

The physician and nursing assessments are combined and a problem list is generated for each applicant. If the physician and nurse disagree about the applicant's ability to live independently, the facility's executive director makes the final decision regarding the person's medical acceptability for admission.

Social Services Assessment. All potential residents are given social services assessments for two purposes: First, to determine if the services (e.g., religious opportunities) provided by the Sunny Acres' community to which they have applied will meet their needs; and, second, to identify any personal interests that may ease adjustment to community life after admission. Once the assessments are completed, an applicant is admitted or denied admittance to the Sunny Acres community.

Data Collection and Management Information

To facilitate management decisions and maximize marketing efforts, an organization must have access to a good information system and database. Currently, however, Sunny Acres' system is somewhat limited, and the limitations are not trivial. To provide a rational basis for accurately predicting future costs and setting its fees, for example, Sunny Acres relies on actuarial analyses, which in turn depend on database integrity for their accuracy.

Sunny Acres' Database Limitations

The major limitation to Sunny Acres' management information system is the absence of health status data such as initial health assessments of residents, or hospital and skilled nursing utilization rates. Thus, links between resident characteristics at initial assessment and services utilization rates, for either individual or aggregate residents, cannot be made. These links provide important analyses to management for guarding against enrolling an adversely selected population, i.e., a population with a higher-than-average probability of requiring costly care.

Data that are available for all current and former residents include:

- sex
- birth date
- entry date to Sunny Acres
- level of care at entry to Sunny Acres
- contract type
- current living status
- date of death
- date of withdrawal from Sunny Acres
- date of transfer to another apartment
- dates of admission and discharge for temporary transfers to a Sunny Acres' skilled nursing facility or to a local hospital
- date of terminal transfer to the skilled nursing facility or hospital.

According to Sunny Acres' chief financial officer, however, the data, in particular the hospital data on many residents, are not always as accurate as they might be.

Actuarial Analysis

Sunny Acres depends on actuarial analyses by consultants to set and determine the adequacy of its fees and to predict future costs, reserve requirements, and service-capacity requirements. Recently, it commissioned studies to determine:

Mortality and Morbidity. Sunny Acres' death and nursing care utilization statistics were compared with those of similar life care communities. The results were used to estimate age/sex-adjusted probabilities of death and nursing home utilization for current and new residents over the next 25 years, and to determine the adequacy of the current number of Sunny Acres' nursing home beds to meet the needs of residents in each of its three communities.

Capital Requirements. Based on projected needs and service costs, Sunny Acres' capital (risk-pool) needs for adequately funding the expected nursing home utilization of current residents were determined.

Pricing Structure. Sunny Acres' current pricing structure for new residents was analyzed against projected utilization and costs to determine its actuarial soundness and capacity to fund expected future costs.

Cash Flow. Finally, pricing and utilization expectations were combined to determine if Sunny Acres' cash flow would be sufficient during the 25 years covered by the projections.

The results of the actuarial studies showed that Sunny Acres has an adequate number of beds system-wide. There were problems, however, with the adequacy of capital to fund the expected nursing home utilization of current residents. Primarily, this lack of capital was due to two factors: First there was insufficient apartment occupancy. A 1981 study, which was the basis for the current rates, had projected 95 percent apartment occupancy by 1986; Sunny Acres had achieved only 83 percent occupancy. Second, monthly fee increases were less than increases in operating expenses (net of depreciation and interest).

The actuaries recommended that monthly fees be increased to at least match increases in operating expenses to ensure Sunny Acres' future financial solvency. They recommended a three percent increase in monthly fees over and above a six percent inflation increase for the subsequent fiscal year. But otherwise, they felt the current pricing structure for new entrants was actuarially sound and, in fact, would create excess funding. They recommended that the excess funding be used to fund an unfunded liability they found associated with current residents.

The actuaries projected that the Denver and Pueblo facilities would have positive cash flows over a ten-year period beginning next year, but the Colorado Springs community would have negative cash flow in year one of that ten-year period. Overall, however, the Sunny Acres system would have a positive cash flow, assuming the Denver and Pueblo units subsidized the Colorado Springs facility.

Problems for Management

The problems faced by Sunny Acres management have varying degrees of complexity. Some are one-time problems or situations that can be resolved satisfactorily with a modicum of time and effort. Others are situational or recurrent, that is, there will be no final resolutions but only strategies for ameliorating the difficulties they cause. Finally, many of them are related; resolving one may exacerbate or alleviate another.

Each of the problems has at least two, sometimes conflicting, perspectives: the organization's and the residents'. And, owing to the nature of a life care community and the contractual agreement between community and resident, resolving them is often an intense—some managers would say "crisis management"—process, requiring a high level of sensitivity to the residents' interests and perceptions.

Questions. The most pressing problems for Sunny Acres are in the areas of admission data collection, occupancy rate and marketing, fee setting, and resident relations. How and in what sequence should management address them? Is there a key problem to the case? If so, what is it?

Admission Data Collection

There is lack of uniform preadmission data collection, particularly in the physician and nursing assessments. For physician assessments, Sunny Acres has no corporate-wide form, such as corporations often use when hiring new employees, for medical examinations. For nursing assessments, there is no system-wide nursing assessment form and no standardized protocol for conducting the assessment. Each Sunny Acres community uses a different instrument to rate applicants. Recently, the chief financial officer's office reviewed random admissions of all residents entering Sunny Acres since 1982 and who later transferred permanently to skilled-nursing beds. Many of the records lacked initial nursing assessment information.

Without uniform and meaningful health status data from admission assessments, linked with subsequent nursing bed utilization data, Sunny Acres' ability to generate timely analyses for fee adjustments and marketing is severely hampered. Also, it heavily weights admission criteria in favor of the applicant's ability to pay

286 / Strategic Planning/Community Relations

current fees (themselves questionable because of the lack of data) rather than on the probability of the applicant using services at a higher-than-average cost later on.

Questions. Correcting this problem will not be a trivial exercise. How should it be approached and where does it begin? How long will it take? How soon will it begin to generate useful information? What other changes or actions will be necessary to maintain the system once it is modified?

Many studies have found that the best demographic indicator of health status for younger adults is social class variously measured by education, occupation, or income. None of these indicators, however, is in Sunny Acres' database. Given the nation's social and economic changes during the last 50 years, is social class an appropriate indicator for persons in the Sunny Acres' age range? If so, which of them should be included in the database?

Occupancy Rate and Marketing

A dramatic decrease in apartment occupancy over the past six years poses a major problem for Sunny Acres, the more so if the trend continues. The rate dropped 12.6 percent: from 95.6 percent in 1983 to 83.0 percent in 1988.

According to Sunny Acres' chief executive officer, the loss of residents is due largely to death. Few move out, and those who do are primarily monthly rather than life care residents. It also appears that residents of apartments have become occupants of nursing beds, and that Sunny Acres' marketing effort has not kept pace with either the death rate or the bed shift.

The three Sunny Acres skilled nursing facilities typically run at more than 90 percent occupancy. In the spring of 1988, for example, the occupancy rate for the Denver facility's 118 beds was 91.5 percent. About 28 percent of the beds were occupied by non-life care residents who pay for their care on a per diem basis. About half of the per diem residents were Medicaid recipients, for whom Colorado Medicaid paid a per diem of $54. The other half were private-pay patients, who paid approximately $70 per day for their care.

But most of the skilled nursing beds (more than 72 percent) are occupied by life care residents. This is a potentially serious fiscal trend for Sunny Acres. Sunny Acres receives no additional reimbursement from life care residents; nursing home care is included in the initial entry and monthly fees.

Declining apartment occupancy has turned marketing into a major activity for Sunny Acres and wrought changes in its marketing strategy, including development of the monthly and capital refund contracts.

It is likely that monthly and capital refund contracts are easier to market than life care contracts. Aside from apartment occupancy, however, a capital refund contract contributes little (10 percent) to Sunny Acres' risk pool and a monthly contract contributes virtually nothing.

Five marketing representatives work under the supervision of a marketing director. They are paid a base salary plus a commission for each contract sold. In 1988, nearly 90 percent of the residents had purchased life care contracts. The recent trend in sales indicates that 50 percent of new purchases are monthly contracts. (Table 14-3).

Sunny Acres' sales staff receive a $750 commission for each life care and capital refund contract sold; the commission is paid when the resident moves in. Commissions for monthly contracts are $250.

Questions. It is not clear whether Sunny Acres management has set restrictions on the mix of residents by contract type, only that all rooms and beds should be filled. Should management set resident mix restrictions? What are the financial risks without restrictions? What are the occupancy rate risks with them?

One way to avoid adverse selection of residents is to practice favorable selection. This means marketing only to persons who present minimal risk probabilities. Should the marketing staff target its sales effort to people with minimal risk characteristics? Would Sunny Acres' mission statement accommodate favorable-selection marketing? Does favorable selection marketing violate the civil rights of potential residents? How else might risk be controlled?

Fee Setting

Sunny Acres' life care entry and monthly fees are set by the chief executive officer and chief financial officer, subject to approval by the board of directors. They are set annually as part of the budgetary process and reflect current and future service costs to the extent that analyses from the database and actuarial studies allow.

Establishing sufficient fees is a difficult task for financial officers. An entry fee should when added to other entry fees, create a risk pool adequate to meet the future costs of providing services to all

Table 14-3 Monthly Marketing Report Sunny Acres Villa, Inc. August 19XX.

	SAV	MED	MDW	VPT	COMBINED	MONTH GOALS	YTD ACTUAL	YTD GOAL
CLOSINGS/MOVE-INS								
Life Care Closings								
Number	1	0	0	2	3	6	7	14
Entry Fees Recieved	$37,775	0	0	$74,985	$112,760			
Monthly Program Move-ins								
Number	5	1	0	0	6	6	11	11
TOTAL	6	1	0	2	9	12	18	25
Actual Move-ins	6	1	0	2	9			
SALES RESULTS (Deposits)								
Life Care Sales (10%)								
Number								
Preferred	1	0	0	0	1	3		
Entry Fees	$57,960	0	0	0	$57,960			
Standard	0	0	0	1	1	2		
Entry Fees	0	0	0	$21,885	$21,885			
Capital Refund	0	0	0	0	0	1		
Entry Fees	0	0	0	0	0			
TOTAL	1	0	0	1	2	6		
Entry Fees	$57,960	0	0	$21,885	$79,845			

Monthly Program (deposits)						
Number	1	2	1	1	5	6
Monthly Prog. Fees	$1,232	$2,249	$515	$682	$4,678	
Total Sales						
(Life Care & Monthly)	2	2	1	2	7	12
Life Care Sales						
Withdrawn/Med Declined	2	1	2	0	5	
OCCUPANCY JULY 19XX						
Occupied Apartments	327	79	101	148	655	649
Reserved Apartments	4	4	2	6	16	16
Available for Sale	83	9	14	1	107	113
Total Apartments	414	92	117	155	778	778
Percentage Occupied	79.0%	85.9%	96.3%	95.5%	84.2%	83.4%
Vacate During Month	1	1	2	1	5	8

Prepared: September 9, 19XX

life care residents; a monthly fee should cover the cash flow and contingency needs of the facility itself while allowing it to remain competitive with the local retirement community marketplace.

Adequate funding of the risk pool may be the most critical issue facing Sunny Acres, particularly if the trend toward monthly contracts continues. Under terms of the life care contract, Sunny Acres assumes considerable long-term risk: It assumes entry fees collected and pooled today will be sufficient to cover the inevitable and unpredictable inflationary increases in skilled nursing and other manpower costs in 5 to 15 or more years. It is obvious, then, that contracts that do not contribute to the risk pool, however much they may improve cash flow, effectively increase the average age (and, hence, the cost) of persons for whom the risk pool is liable. Further complicating the matter, the persons for whom the risk pool is liable may be admitted at a younger age, quite possibly for an entry fee below current price. It is a dilemma not unlike that facing the Social Security system, which is now paying many beneficiaries more in a year than they contributed during their entire working life.

Questions. The actuaries found the $50,000 entry fee presently adequate to cover cost contingencies over a remaining life span of new life care residents. Actuarial analysis, however, is an imprecise science, usually relying on age/sex-adjusted (but neither social-class nor medical-exam adjusted) experience data from more or less similar organizations. How can management assure itself that the actuarial estimates are efficacious for Sunny Acres' financial health?

The actuaries also found that two of Sunny Acres' three communities would have positive cash flow but the third would have negative cash flow in the years ahead. Assuming that the three communities operate at the same level of efficiency, should the surplus revenue from the positive-flow communities cover the losses of the negative-flow community? If not, how should the losses be covered and what should the surplus funds be used for?

Resident Relations

Harmonious relations among residents and between residents and management are critical to the success and survival of Sunny Acres' life care communities. Because the life care residents are self-selected and have similar personal characteristics, their preferences and attitudes are likely to conflict with those of monthly paying and capital refund residents. Also, the characteristics of life care residents combine to create, among other things, an expectation of accountability from management. They perceive themselves as participating investors and decision-making customers, rather than passive tenants or patients. Decisions made by management, from price increases to repainting halls, will be scrutinized and disputed by residents demanding explanations and justifications.

In the recent past, relations between residents and management at Sunny Acres have been marked by distrust. This situation indicates that there is ineffective communication between them which causes some residents to perceive management as disinterested in their concerns. In some instances, relations deteriorated to the point where groups of residents had retained attorneys to protect their interests and to represent them in complaints filed with regulatory agencies against Sunny Acres.

Questions. Mission statements are how organizations define themselves and their social commitment to their clients. Can Sunny Acres' management problems be resolved adequately within the philosophic boundaries of its mission statement? Sunny Acres' consultants have recommended expansion of services beyond skilled-nursing care to appeal to a younger population. Is this suggestion germane to the current problems? If so, what services should be added and for which age groups? Should the new services be available to the current residents also? If so, how should the financial risk be controlled? If not, how should resident relations be handled?